Weight Gain C

For Beginners

50+ Delicious Recipes and Simple Strategies to Pack on Pounds and Build Muscle Mass

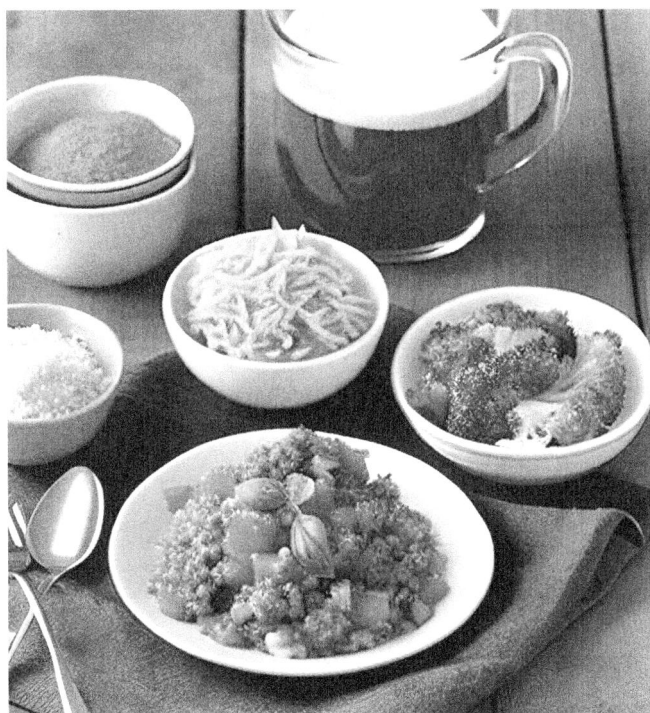

Rachel Carter

Table of Contents

CONCLUSION

14-DAYS WEIGHT GAIN PLANNER

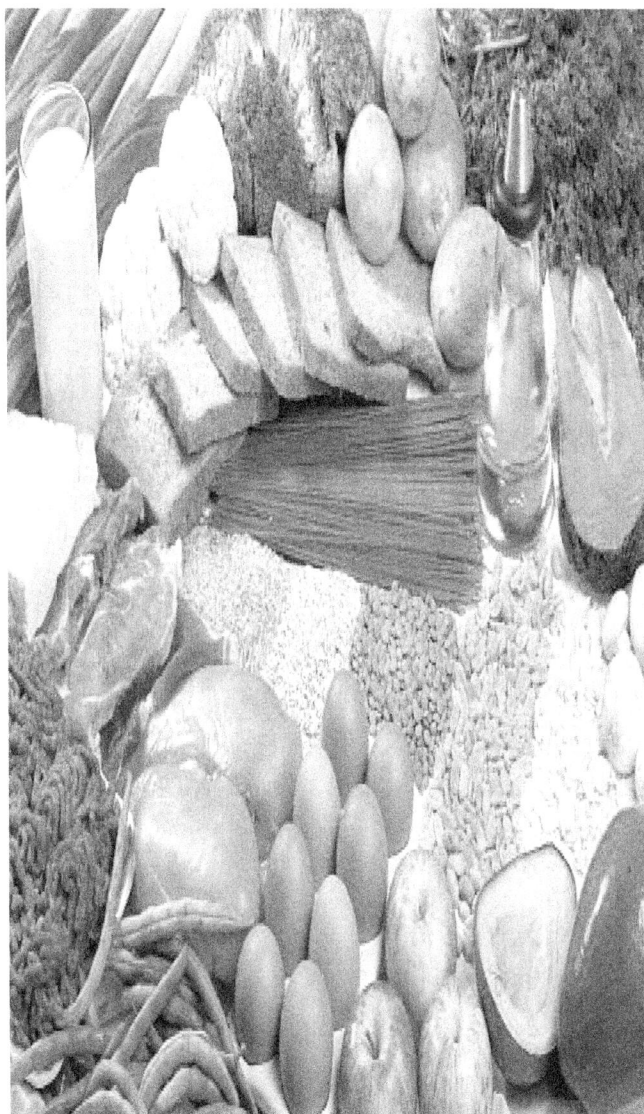

INTRODUCTION

Elizabeth has always had a thin build. She loved delicious food, but she never appeared to put on any weight. Elizabeth, however, became aware that her metabolism was slowing down as she reached her thirties and that she was finding it difficult to maintain her weight. Previously, she had never given much thought to gaining weight, but at this time, she was tempted to do so.

Elizabeth started looking into healthy ways to gain weight, and she soon found that it was all about the food she consumed. She needed to eat more calories each day than she expended, and she wanted to accomplish it in a way that was both healthy for her body and sustainable.

When she did, a beginner's cookbook for weight gain was the ideal remedy. She might gain weight in a healthy way thanks to the cookbook's many scrumptious and nutritious dishes.

Elizabeth was eager to test out the recipes and see whether they could assist her in gaining weight.

She started with the morning meals, which included lots of foods strong in protein and smoothies with lots of calories. She adored the spinach and feta egg scramble as well as the blueberry protein pancakes. She was able to begin her day with a filling and tasty supper because they were simple to prepare.

Elizabeth discovered a variety of options for lunch and dinner. The cookbook included everything from grilled chicken and vegetable skewers to hearty stews and casseroles. She likes the diversity of choices and could always find something to satisfy her mood or cravings. Even vegan and vegetarian options proved to be surprisingly satisfying and delectable.

Elizabeth began to observe changes in her body as she worked her way through the cookbook.

She felt stronger and more energized, and her clothes fit a little better. She continued to prepare wholesome, nourishing meals from the cookbook since she was happy with her progress.

Yet, there were obstacles in the road. Elizabeth periodically found it difficult to consume enough calories to satisfy her calorie targets, and she occasionally discovered that she was reaching for unhealthy treats out of habit. She was determined to stick to her plan and gain the weight she had set out to.

Elizabeth was able to gain the weight she desired using the recipes in a healthy and sustainable way. She carried on preparing tasty and wholesome meals from the cookbook, and she was pleased with the development she had made. Elizabeth had learned that gaining weight required proper nutrition and healthful lifestyle choices in addition to binging on junk food and engaging in other unhealthy vices.

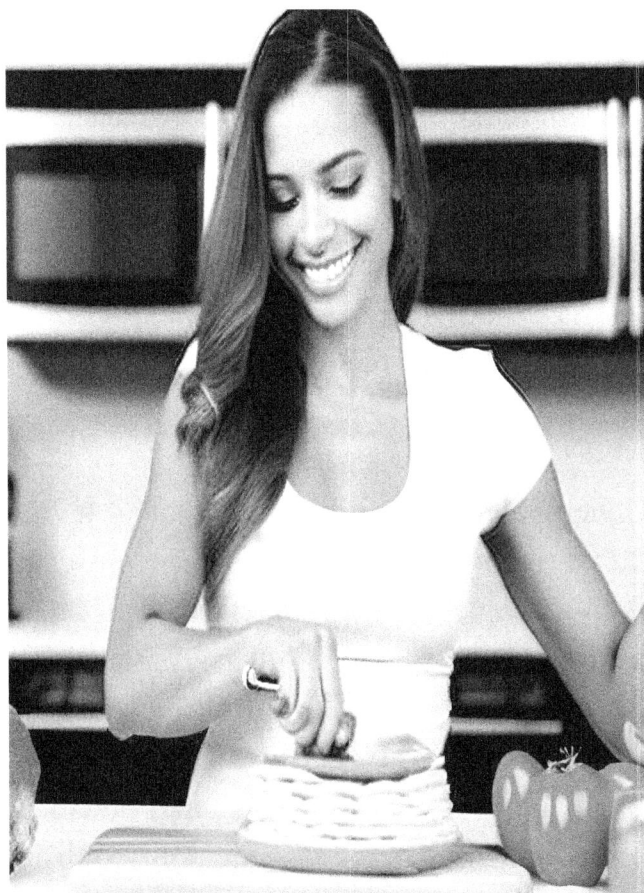

CHAPTER ONE

Definition of Weight Gain

Weight gain is a word used to describe the process of gaining weight, usually as a result of body fat accumulating. Those who are underweight or have a low body mass index frequently find it to be a desirable objective (BMI). But, weight gain can also happen accidentally and may indicate an underlying medical issue.

Genetics, diet, and lifestyle are just a few of the variables that might affect weight gain. Some people can be genetically prone to gaining weight, while others might suffer with weight growth as a result of inactivity or a poor diet. Weight gain can also be caused by specific drugs and medical disorders, such as hypothyroidism, Cushing's disease, and polycystic ovarian syndrome (PCOS).

The most typical strategy for gaining weight on purpose is to eat more calories while keeping or raising physical activity levels. A diet rich in nutrient-dense foods, such as lean protein, whole grains, fruits, and vegetables, can help you achieve this. To help them reach their weight-gain objectives, some people additionally include high-calorie meals and supplements in their diet, like protein smoothies and weight-gain powders.

It's crucial to remember, though, that weight increase should always be addressed in a sustainable and healthy way. For example, Fast weight gain and excessive calorie consumption can have a severe impact on health, increasing the risk of diabetes and heart disease.While starting a weight gain journey, it's crucial to collaborate with a medical expert or certified nutritionist to make sure that goals are reasonable and healthy.

Gaining weight may have psychological effects as well, especially in a culture where being slim is frequently associated with attractiveness and desirability. Some people could experience self-esteem and body image problems as a result of weight increase, and they might find counseling or support groups helpful in addressing these difficulties.

In conclusion, gaining weight is a difficult process that is affected by several variables. Individuals can reach their weight gain goals while maintaining their general health and wellness by working with a healthcare expert and addressing any potential psychological ramifications.

Why Gaining Weight is Important for You.

For those who are underweight or have a low BMI, gaining weight might be a major objective.Although society frequently advocates thinness as the ideal body type, being underweight can really have detrimental effects on one's health. Here are a few explanations as to why gaining weight can be crucial for you:

A healthy body weight serves to encourage the generation of immune cells that fight off infections and disease, which is why it is linked to increased immune function.

Improved energy levels: The body needs a sufficient amount of calories to power everyday activities and maintain energy levels. Those who are underweight could experience weariness or struggle to execute physical duties.

Improved mental health: Those who are underweight may be more susceptible to anxiety, depression, and other mental health problems. Increasing weight and getting to a healthy body weight might enhance one's mood and mental state generally.

Decreased risk of osteoporosis: Osteoporosis, a disorder that weakens bones and makes patients more prone to fractures, can be brought on by low body weight. Getting to a healthy weight can aid in lowering this risk.

Enhanced fertility: Women who are underweight may experience difficulties getting pregnant since low body weight might mess with their hormones and menstrual cycles. Putting on weight can boost fertility and balance hormones.

Gaining weight can aid in gaining muscle mass, which is essential for general strength and athletic performance. A healthy diet and resistance training can support muscular growth.

Enhanced general health: Keeping a healthy weight is linked to a lower risk of chronic conditions like heart disease, diabetes, and some malignancies. Healthy

and sustainable weight gain can lower the risk of disease and
enhance overall health.

It's crucial to remember that gaining weight should always be done so in a healthy and sustainable fashion, with the help of a trained dietician or healthcare provider.Fast weight growth or consuming too many calories can have a detrimental impact on one's health and may not be the best way to acquire weight over the long term.

To sum up, for people who are underweight or have a low BMI, gaining weight might be an important aim. The immune system, energy levels, mental health, fertility, muscle mass, and general health can all be enhanced by achieving a healthy body weight. Yet, it's crucial to approach weight growth in a sustainable and healthy way, with advice from a healthcare provider.

Understanding Macronutrients and Their Role in Weight Gain

Macronutrients are the essential components of our diet that provide us with energy, and understanding their role in weight gain is crucial for those looking to increase their body weight. The three main macronutrients are carbohydrates, proteins, and fats, and each plays a different role in the body.

The body uses carbohydrates as its main source of energy, which are present in foods including grains, fruits, and vegetables. When consumed, carbohydrates are converted to glucose and released into the circulation, where they are used as energy by the body's cells. An energy boost from consuming a diet rich in carbohydrates is beneficial for people trying to put on weight and build muscle.

Proteins are essential for the growth and repair of the body's tissues, including muscle tissue. They are found in foods such as meat, fish, dairy products, and legumes. As protein is consumed, it is converted into amino acids, which are then utilized by the body to create and repair tissues. A diet rich in protein is essential for people trying to gain weight since it helps support muscle growth and repair.

Fats have a crucial role in the storage of energy, insulation, and defense of key organs. They can be found in foods including nuts, seeds, oils, and fatty seafood. After being consumed, fats are converted into fatty acids and kept in the body's adipose tissue. A diet rich in beneficial fats, like monounsaturated and polyunsaturated fats, can encourage weight gain and good health in general.

Understanding how macronutrients impact weight gain is essential because it enables people to tailor their diets to meet their unique needs. Those who want to gain weight and grow muscle, for example, may benefit from a diet high in protein and carbohydrates, while those who wish to maintain their weight may benefit from a diet high in healthy fats.

It's crucial to remember that the type of macronutrients consumed affects both general health and weight growth. A diet heavy in processed carbs, saturated fats, and unhealthy proteins may not be the best choice for promoting weight growth and can have detrimental effects on health.

How To Use This Cookbook

A weight gain cookbook can help you reach your weight gain objectives and enhance your general health. But, especially for novices, navigating through the recipes and meal planning can be intimidating. The following advice will help you use a weight gain cookbook to get the outcomes you want:

Learn the recipes: Before you begin to cook, spend some time reading the recipes to acquire a sense of the ingredients and preparation techniques used. You can use this to organize your meals and make sure you have all the supplies on hand.

Arrange your meals: Utilizing a cookbook for weight gain can be a fantastic way to organize your menus and make sure you're eating a healthy, balanced diet. Plan your meals carefully for the coming week, including a mix of macronutrients and foods that are high in nutrients.

Check your progress: Monitoring your weight gain will help you stay motivated and make sure you are on the right path to achieving your objectives. Track your meals, calories consumed, and rate of weight gain over time using a food diary or an app.

Try multiple recipes: Don't be hesitant to experiment with new dishes, ingredients,

and cooking techniques. This can assist in keeping meals interesting and avoiding boredom, which is often a
barrier to successful weight gain.

Including physical activity: Physical activity is crucial for weight gain and overall health in addition to a balanced diet. Strength training and other physical activities should be a part of your routine to encourage muscle growth and enhance general health.

Consult a professional: It's vital to seek advice from a certified dietician or healthcare provider if you have specific health problems or concerns about weight gain. They may assist you in creating a specialized weight gain plan that is catered to your particular requirements and objectives.

Finally, employing a weight gain cookbook can help you reach your weight gain objectives and enhance your general health.

You may optimize your results and reach your targeted weight gain outcomes by being familiar with the recipes, planning your meals, keeping track of your progress, trying out different recipes, including physical activity, and getting professional advice.

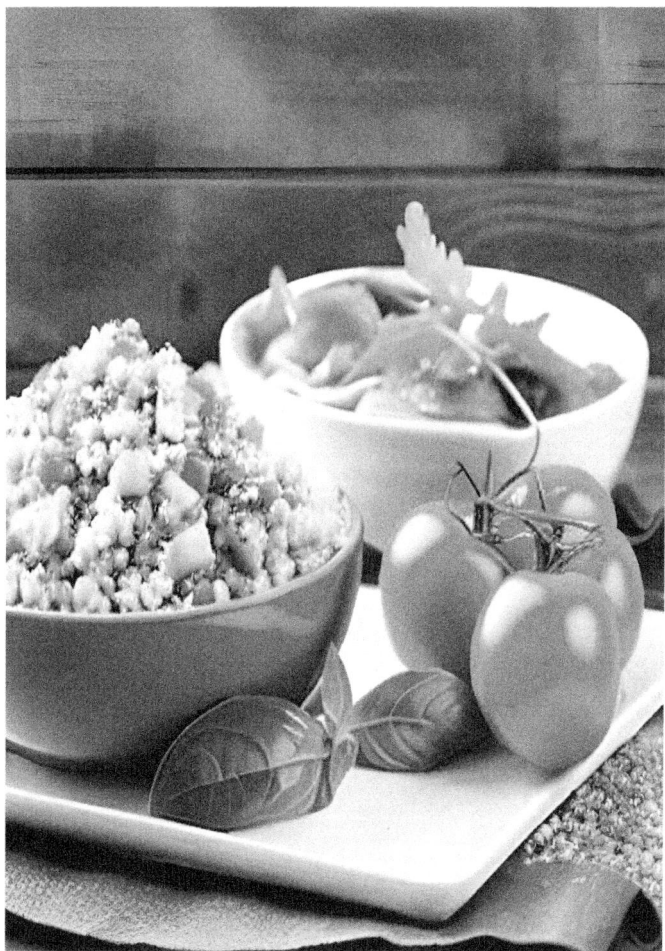

CHAPTER TWO

Planning for Weight Gain

Preparation is an essential step in reaching any goal, and gaining weight is no different. Planning is really significantly more important when trying to gain weight because it requires making major dietary and lifestyle adjustments. Beginners will learn the significance of planning ahead for weight gain in this chapter, which also offers advice and techniques for creating a successful weight gain strategy. Readers will obtain a thorough grasp of what it takes to develop a successful weight gain plan and position themselves for long-term success, from setting realistic goals to spotting potential hurdles.

Setting Realistic Goals For Weight Gain

Anyone trying to gain weight in a healthy and sustainable manner must set realistic goals. When it comes to weight gain, it's crucial to take a long-term perspective and concentrate on making slow, steady progress rather than hoping to see results right away. This section will cover the significance of setting reasonable goals as well as practical advice on how to do so.

Understanding what is feasible and healthy for your body is the first step in establishing realistic weight gain objectives. While eating a lot of high-calorie foods will cause you to gain weight quickly, this strategy is unsustainable and can eventually have a negative impact on your health.Instead, strive for a weekly weight gain of 1-2 pounds, which is seen to be a healthy and doable amount.

Secondly, think about your present diet and lifestyle practices. Setting objectives that are realistic for your current circumstances is crucial. For instance, switching overnight to a diet heavy in calories and protein may be impossible if you are currently following a low-calorie, low-protein diet. Set manageable objectives instead, like increasing the amount of protein in each meal or including a protein smoothie into your daily routine.

It's crucial to take into account any obstacles or difficulties you might face while trying to acquire weight.for instance, it could be difficult to consistently consume adequate calories and protein if your busy schedule leaves little time for meal preparation. Setting realistic goals in this situation can entail locating quick and convenient food options that work with your schedule, including meal preparation on the weekends or keeping wholesome snacks on hand.

Monitoring your progress and making any necessary adjustments to your goals is another crucial component of setting realistic objectives. You may find out where you might need to make changes by keeping track of your protein and calorie consumption as well as your weight on a regular basis. For instance, you might need to raise your calorie consumption or change your macronutrient intake if you are not experiencing the required weight growth after many weeks.

Calculating Daily Calorie Needs

Planning to gain weight requires making a daily calorie needs calculation. Your body needs a certain number of calories each day to maintain your weight and carry out your daily tasks. These calories are known as your daily caloric needs. You must consume more calories daily than your body expels in order to gain weight. We'll go through how to figure out how many calories you need each day in this section, along with some advice on how to change your diet to gain weight.

You must first ascertain your basal metabolic rate (BMR) in order to calculate your daily calorie requirements. Your body consumes calories during rest to support essential processes like breathing and circulation, which is measured as BMR. BMR can be calculated using a number of different formulas, but the Harris-Benedict equation is the most popular one. Your age, height, weight, and gender are all factors in this equation.

Your activity level must be taken into account after calculating your BMR in order to compute your daily energy expenditure (TDEE). TDEE is the total daily energy expenditure, which includes calories burned through physical activity. There are several ways to gauge activity level, including the categories of Sedentary, Lightly Active, Moderately Active, Very Active, and

Extremely Active.

After determining your TDEE, you can increase this figure by 250–500 calories to produce the calorie excess required for weight gain. If your TDEE is 2,000 calories, for instance, you should try to eat 2,250–2,500 calories daily to gain weight.

It's crucial to remember that everyone has varied caloric needs, which might change depending on things like heredity, hormones, and lifestyle. Also, it's critical to modify your calorie intake as you put on weight because your body weight will cause an increase in your calorie requirements.

It's essential to track your calorie intake and modify your diet as necessary to make sure you are getting enough calories to gain weight. Given that it offers recipes and meal plans intended to help you meet your weight gain objectives, the weight gain cookbook for beginners might be a useful tool in this situation. Adding calorie-dense items like almonds, nut butter, avocados, and dried fruit to your diet will also help you consume more calories without eating more food.

Planning Meals And Snacks For Weight Gain

Gaining weight requires careful planning of meals and snacks. You must consume more calories than your body burns each day if you want to acquire weight. Yet, increasing caloric intake alone is insufficient. To encourage healthy weight gain, it's crucial to concentrate on nutrient-dense meals and develop a balanced diet. This part will cover planning advice for meals and snacks to promote weight gain as well as how the weight gain cookbook for beginners can support your objectives.

The macronutrient balance of your diet should be taken into account while planning meals and snacks for weight gain. The three macronutrients are fat, protein, and carbs.Each of these is essential to how your body works and should be consumed in the right quantities.

As they make up the majority of your calorie consumption, carbohydrates should be your main source of energy. Excellent sources of complex carbs that give you energy and critical nutrients are whole grains, fruits, and vegetables.

Building and rebuilding muscle tissue, which is critical for weight growth, requires protein. Lean meats, poultry, fish, eggs, dairy products, legumes, and nuts are all excellent sources of protein.

Moreover, fat is a necessary ingredient that stimulates the creation of hormones, gives us energy, and aids in vitamin absorption. Your diet should contain healthy fats such those in avocados, nuts, seeds, and olive oil.

Aim to include a range of nutrient-dense foods from each macronutrient group when preparing your meals and snacks. The beginner's weight gain cookbook can be a useful resource for organizing wholesome meals and snacks that promote healthy weight gain. A balance of carbohydrates, protein, and fat is included in the cookbook's recipes and meal plans.

It's vital to balance macronutrients while also taking meal frequency and portion sizes into account. You can enhance your calorie intake and support weight growth by eating several smaller, more frequent meals and snacks throughout the day. Choose calorie-dense items like nuts, dried fruit, and high-calorie smoothies to eat around every two to three hours.

It's crucial to pay attention to your body when it comes to portion sizes and eat until you are completely satisfied. But, if you're having trouble reaching your calorie targets, it could be necessary to boost your portion sizes or include more snacks.

Understanding Portion Sizes And Serving Recommendations

The size of your portions matters when it comes to gaining weight. Eating too little or too much can impede your progress or result in unhealthful weight gain. Making informed decisions and achieving your weight gain objectives healthily can be facilitated by having a solid understanding of serving sizes and recommended portions.

Using visual clues is one approach to comprehend portion sizes. A serving of fat, for instance, should be around the size of your thumb, a serving of protein, roughly the size of your palm, and a serving of carbohydrates, roughly the size of your fist. You can ensure that you are getting enough of each macronutrient by using these visual clues to help you determine the proper portion proportions.

Using measuring implements, such as a food scale or measuring cups, is a further technique to comprehend portion amounts. By measuring your meals, you may ensure that you aren't unintentionally overestimating or underestimating your calorie intake and have a better understanding of proper portion proportions.

It's essential to pay attention to the serving suggestions given in each recipe when utilizing the weight gain cookbook for beginners. These portions are made to help you reach your calorie targets and guarantee a macronutrient consumption that is balanced. Increase meal sizes or include more snacks throughout the day if you're having trouble reaching your calorie targets.

The quality of the foods you eat should also be taken into account in addition to portion amounts. Choosing nutrient-dense foods, such as fruits, vegetables, lean meats, and healthy fats, will help you stay healthy. These foods supply important macronutrients, vitamins, and minerals that support a healthy increase in body weight. The timing of your meals and snacks is another crucial factor. Your calorie intake can be increased and weight growth supported by eating several smaller, more frequent meals and snacks throughout the day. Attempt to eat every two to three hours, and select calorie-dense meals like almonds, dried fruit, and smoothies with lots of calories.

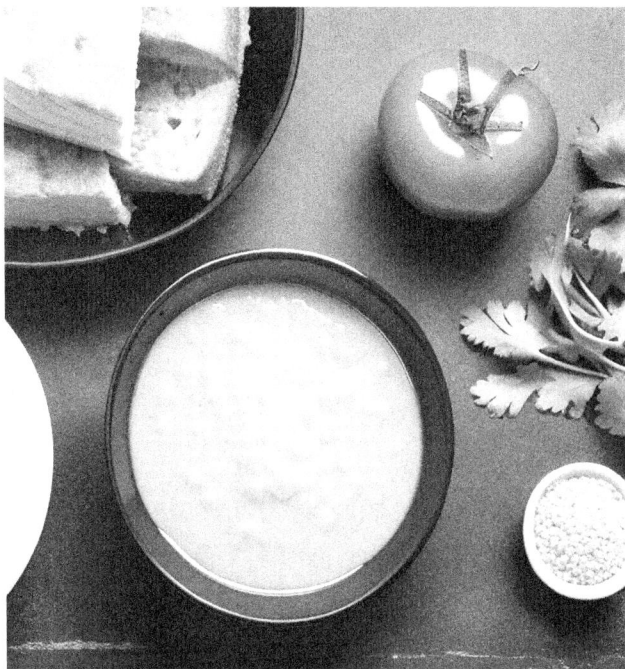

CHAPTER THREE

Breakfast Recipes

High-Calorie Smoothies And Shakes

High-calorie smoothies and shakes can be a great option for those looking to gain weight or add some extra calories to their diet. Not only are they easy to prepare, but they also offer a wide variety of flavors and ingredients to choose from. In this piece, we will explore some delicious and nutritious smoothie and shake recipes that you can try for your breakfast.

Ingredients:

• 1 large banana (approximately 121g)
• 2 tbsp of Peanut Butter (approximately 32g)
• 1/2 cup of greek yoghurt (approximately 113g)

•1 cup of whole Milk (approximately 240ml)
•1 tbsp of honey (approximately 21g)
•1 tsp of vanilla Extract (approximately 5ml)

Method of Preparation:

1. Start by slicing the banana into small pieces after peeling it.

2. Combine the pieces of banana, 2 tablespoons of peanut butter, 1/2 cup of Greek yogurt, 1 cup of whole milk, 1 tablespoon of honey, and 1 teaspoon of vanilla extract in a blender.

3. Combine all the ingredients in a blender and process until they have a smooth, creamy consistency.

4. Pour the mixture into a tall glass, and then savor your delectable smoothie with lots of calories!

You might also try this recipe for a calorie-dense shake:

Ingredients:

- 1/2 cup (approximately 40g) of Oats
- 2 scoops (approximately 30g) of Chocolate
- Protein Powder
- 2 tbsp (approximately 32g) of Peanut Butter
- 1 cup (approximately 240ml) of Whole Milk
- 4-5 Ice Cubes

Method of Preparation:

1. To begin, add 1/2 cup of oats to a blender and process until a fine powder is obtained.

2. Fill the blender with 1 cup of whole milk, 4-5 ice cubes, 2 scoops of chocolate protein powder, 2 tablespoons of peanut butter, and all of these ingredients.

3. Combine all the ingredients in a blender and process until they have a smooth, creamy consistency.

4. Pour the mixture into a tall glass, then savor your tasty, calorie-dense shake!

These delectable, high-calorie shakes and smoothies are also nutrient-rich and can aid in your weight-gain objectives. The oats and chocolate protein powder shake provides a wonderful mix of carbohydrates, while the banana and peanut butter smoothie is a fantastic source of protein, healthy fats, and carbohydrates

Pancakes And Waffles

Pancakes and waffles are two classic breakfast foods that can be a great option for those looking to gain weight. Not only are they easy to make, but they also offer a delicious and satisfying way to add some extra calories to your diet.

Ingredients:

Pancakes:

• 1 cup of all purpose flour (approximately 120g)
• 1 tsp of baking powder (approximately 5g)
• 1/4 tsp of salt (approximately 1g)
• 2 tbsp of granulated sugar (approximately 25g)
• 1 cup of whole milk (approximately 240ml)
• 1 large egg
• 2 tbsp of unsalted butter (approximately 30g)

Method of Preparation:

1. Combine 1 cup of all-purpose flour, 1 teaspoon of baking powder, 1/4 teaspoon of salt, and 2 tablespoons of granulated sugar in a mixing bowl.

2. Combine 1 cup of whole milk, 1 large egg, and 2 tablespoons of melted unsalted butter in another mixing bowl.

3. Combine the dry ingredients by adding the wet ingredients and stirring just until combined. Do not overmix the batter.

4. Put a nonstick pan on the stovetop at medium heat. As soon as bubbles start to appear on the surface, pour 1/4 cup of the batter into the pan and fry it. The pancake should turn golden brown after another minute of cooking.

5. Carry out step 5 with the remaining batter.

Waffles:

• 1 1/2 cups of all-purpose flour (approximately 180g)
• 2 tsp of baking powder (approximately 10g)
• 1/2 tsp of salt (approximately 2g)
• 2 tbsp of granulated sugar(approximately 25g)
• 1 cup of whole milk(approximately 240ml)
• 2 large eggs

•1/2 cup of unsalted butter(approximately 113g), melted

•1 tsp of vanilla extract (approximately 5ml)

Method of Preparation:

1. Add 2 tbsp of granulated sugar, 1 1/2 cups of all-purpose flour, 2 tsp of baking powder, and 1/2 tsp of salt to a mixing bowl.

2. Combine 1/2 cup of melted unsalted butter, 1 teaspoon of vanilla extract, 1 cup of whole milk, 2 large eggs, and 1/2 cup in another mixing bowl.

3. Stir the dry ingredients just enough to combine after adding the wet ingredients. You shouldn't overmix the batter.

4. As per the directions from the manufacturer, preheat your waffle maker. Onto each waffle grid, pour 1/4 cup of the batter, and bake until crisp and golden.

5. Add any desired garnishes, such as fresh fruit, whipped cream, or syrup, to the pancakes or waffles before serving.

These pancake and waffle recipes are a delicious and easy way to add some extra calories to your breakfast. The pancake recipe offers a fluffy and light texture, while the waffle recipe gives you a crispy and golden brown exterior. Both recipes are versatile and can be customized with your favorite toppings and flavors. So why not give them a try and enjoy a satisfying and filling breakfast?

Oatmeal And Porridge Variations

Oatmeal and porridge are popular breakfast choices that can help you gain weight. They are nutritious, filling, and easy to customize with a variety of ingredients. In this writing, we will explore some delicious oatmeal and porridge variations that you can try for your breakfast.

Oatmeal

Ingredients:

- 1 cup of rolled oats (approximately 90g)
- 2 cups of water (approximately 480ml)
- 1 cup of whole milk (approximately 240ml)
- 2 tbsp of brown milk (approximately 25g)
- 1 tsp of cinnamon powder (approximately 5g)
- 1/4 cup of Chopped Nuts such as almonds, walnuts, or pecans.(approximately 30g)

Method of Preparation:

1. Bring 2 cups of water to a boil in a saucepan. Turn the heat down to low and add 1 cup of rolled oats.

2. Cook the oats for 10 to 15 minutes, or until they are tender and have absorbed most of the liquid, stirring occasionally.

3. Combine the oats with 1 cup of whole milk, 2 tablespoons of brown sugar, and 1 teaspoon of cinnamon powder. Stir thoroughly to mix.

4. Continue to cook the oats for an additional 2 to 3 minutes, or until they reach the consistency you prefer.

5. Arrange the oats in bowls and sprinkle chopped nuts on top.

Porridge:

Ingredients:

• 1 cup of rolled oats (approximately 90g)
• 2 cups of water(approximately 480ml)
• 1 cup of whole milk (approximately 240ml)
• 1/4 tsp of salt (approximately 1g)
• 2 tbsp of honey (approximately 25g)
• 1/4 cup of Dried Fruits such as raisins, cranberries, or apricots (approximately 30g)

Method of Preparation:

1. Heat two cups of water to a rolling boil in a saucepan. Turn down the heat, then stir in 1 cup of rolled oats.

2. Cook the oats for 10 to 15 minutes, or until they have absorbed the majority of the liquid and are tender.

3. Add 2 tbsp of honey, 1 cup of whole milk, and 1/4 teaspoon of salt to the oats. Mix thoroughly by stirring.

4. Once the porridge has the consistency you prefer, cook the oats for an additional 2 to 3 minutes.

5. Arrange bowls with the porridge and top with dried fruit.

Breakfast Sandwiches And Wraps

Breakfast sandwiches and wraps are a convenient and tasty way to start your day.

They can be packed with protein and carbohydrates to help you gain weight and stay full until your next meal.

Breakfast Sandwich

Ingredients:

- 1 Whole wheat English muffin or bagel
- 2-3 slices of Cooked sausage or bacon
- 2 Scrambled eggs
- 1 slice Cheddar cheese
- Salt and pepper to taste
- Butter or oil for cooking

Method of Preparation:

1. Slice the bagel or English muffin in half, then lightly toast each half until golden.

2. In a skillet, crisp up the sausage or bacon. Take out and place aside.

3. Scramble the eggs in the same skillet with a tablespoon of butter or oil.

Add salt and pepper to taste.

4. After the eggs have finished cooking, top them with a slice of cheddar cheese and let it melt.

5. Put the toasted English muffin or bagel on top of the cooked sausage or bacon to assemble the sandwich. Then top with cheese-topped scrambled eggs. Cover with the bagel or English muffin's top half.

Breakfast Wrap

Ingredients:

- •1 Whole wheat tortilla
- •2-3 slices of Cooked turkey or ham
- •2 Scrambled eggs
- •1/4 Avocado
- •1/4 cup of Spinach leaves
- •Salt and pepper to taste
- •Butter or oil for cooking

Method of Preparation:

1. Heat the turkey or ham thoroughly in a skillet. Take out and place aside.

2. Scramble the eggs with a tablespoon of butter or oil in the same skillet. Add salt and pepper to taste.

3. After the eggs are done cooking, remove them from the skillet and sanitize it.

4. Slice the avocado's flesh after cutting it in half, then remove the pit.

5. In the same skillet, heat the tortilla until it becomes slightly crispy.

6. Put the warmed tortilla on a plate and put together the wrap. Add the cooked turkey or ham, beaten eggs, and avocado slices after the spinach leaves. Add extra salt and pepper if desired.

These breakfast sandwich and wrap recipes are easy to make and can be customized with your favorite ingredients. They are perfect for busy mornings when you need a quick and filling meal to start your day. The breakfast sandwich offers a classic and savory taste, while the breakfast wrap provides a fresh and light flavor.

Egg dishes

Eggs are a staple breakfast food that can be used to create a variety of delicious and healthy dishes. They are packed with protein and nutrients that can help you gain weight and maintain a healthy body. In this article, we will explore some delicious egg dishes that you can try for your next breakfast.

Scrambled Eggs

Ingredients:

•2 Eggs
•Butter or oil for cooking
•Salt and pepper to taste

Method of Preparation:

2. In a bowl, whisk the eggs until they are fluffy. Add a little salt and pepper, then completely combine.

2. Melt a tablespoon of butter or oil in a nonstick skillet over medium heat.

3. Place the skillet over medium heat and add the beaten eggs. The eggs should be gently scrambled with a spatula until they are fully done.

4. Present warm with toast or a serving of fruit.

Omelette

Ingredients:

•2-3 Eggs
•Butter or oil for cooking
•Salt and pepper to taste
•1/4 cup of Cheddar cheese

- 1/4 cup of Ham or sausage
- 1/4 cup of Spinach leaves

Method of Preparation:

1. Beat the eggs in a bowl until they are fluffy. Mix thoroughly after adding a touch of salt and pepper.

2. Melt a tablespoon of butter or oil in a nonstick skillet over medium heat.

3. Place the skillet over medium heat and add the beaten eggs. Lift the omelette's edges with a spatula to let the raw eggs fall to the bottom of the skillet.

4. After the eggs have set, top one side of the omelette with cheese, ham or sausage, and spinach leaves.

5. Fold the other side of the omelette over the filling using a spatula.

6. Continue cooking for one more minute, or until the cheese has melted and the filling is thoroughly heated.

7. Serve hot with toast or a side of fruit.

Frittata

Ingredients:

•6 Eggs
•Butter or oil for cooking
•Salt and pepper to taste
•1/4 cup of Cheddar cheese
•1/4 cup of Ham or sausage
•1/4 cup of Broccoli
•1/4 of Red bell pepper

Method of Preparation:

1. Set the oven's temperature to 350°F.

2. Beat the eggs in a bowl until they are fluffy. Mix thoroughly after adding a touch of salt and pepper.

3. Melt a tablespoon of butter or oil in a sizable oven-safe skillet.

4. Add the broccoli, red bell pepper, and ham or sausage to the skillet and cook for 5 minutes.

5. After adding the vegetables evenly with a spatula, pour the beaten eggs into the skillet.

6. Top the eggs with some cheddar cheese.

7. Bake the skillet in the oven for 15-20 minutes, or until the cheese is melted and the eggs are set.

8. Warm up and serve with toast or a side of fruit.

These egg recipes are simple to prepare and are adaptable to your preferred additions. These are ideal for hectic mornings when you need a quick meal that will fill you up and get your day started. While the omelette and frittata offer a more sophisticated and rich taste, scrambled eggs offer a more traditional and straightforward flavor.

Breakfast Casseroles And Bake

Breakfast casseroles and bakes are hearty and filling dishes that are perfect for those looking to gain weight in a healthy way. They are versatile and can be made with a variety of ingredients, making them a great option for those who like to mix things up in the kitchen. In this writing, we will explore some delicious breakfast casserole and bake recipes that you can try for your next breakfast.

Sausage Breakfast Casserole

Ingredients:

- 1 lb of Ground breakfast sausage
- 6 slices, cubed Bread
- 6 Eggs
- 2 cups Milk
- 1 cup, shredded Cheddar cheese
- Salt and pepper to taste

•Butter for greasing the casserole dish

Method of Preparation:

1. Preheat the oven to 350°F.

2. In a skillet, cook the breakfast sausage over medium heat until browned and cooked through.

3. Grease a 9x13 inch casserole dish with butter. Place the cubed bread in the bottom of the dish.

4. Combine the milk and eggs in a bowl. Mix thoroughly after adding a touch of salt and pepper.

5. Cover the bread in the casserole dish with the egg mixture. Top the egg mixture with the cooked sausage.

6. Top the casserole with the cheddar cheese that has been shredded.

7. Bake for 35 to 40 minutes in a preheated oven, or until the cheese is melted and bubbling and the eggs are set.

8. Serve hot and enjoy!

Hash Brown Breakfast Bake

Ingredients:

•30 oz Frozen hash browns
•6 Eggs
•1 cup of Milk
•2 cup, shredded Cheddar cheese
•6 slices, cooked and crumbled Bacon
•1/4 cup, chopped Green onions
•Salt and pepper to taste
•Butter for greasing the casserole dish

Method of Preparation:

1. Preheat the oven to 350°F.

2. Grease a 9x13 inch casserole dish with butter.

Spread the frozen hash browns evenly in the bottom of the dish.

3. Combine the eggs and milk in a bowl. Mix thoroughly after adding a touch of salt and pepper.

4. In the casserole dish with the hash browns, pour the egg mixture over them.

5. Top the egg mixture with the shredded cheddar cheese, crumbled bacon, and finely chopped green onions.

6. Bake in the preheated oven for 40-45 minutes, or until the eggs are set and the cheese is melted and bubbly.

7. Serve hot and enjoy!

These breakfast casseroles and bakes are perfect for feeding a crowd or for meal prep. They can be customized to suit your taste preferences and can be made ahead of time, making them a great option for busy mornings.

Muffins And Breads

Muffins and breads are a delicious and easy way to incorporate nutritious ingredients into your breakfast routine. Whether you prefer sweet or savory, there are countless varieties to choose from that can help you gain weight in a healthy way. In this writing, we will explore some delicious muffin and bread recipes that you can try for your next breakfast.

Blueberry Muffins

Ingredients:

- 2 cups of All-purpose flour
- 2 tsp of Baking powder
- 1/2 tsp of Salt
- 3/4 cup of White sugar
- 2 Eggs
- 1/2 cup of Milk
- 1/2 cup of Vegetable oil

•1 1/2 cups, fresh or frozen Blueberries

Method of Preparation:

1. Preheat the oven to 375°F.

2. Combine the flour, baking powder, salt, and sugar in a sizable mixing bowl. Mix thoroughly.

3. Beat the eggs in a separate bowl. Mix well after adding the milk and vegetable oil.

4. Combine the dry ingredients with the wet ingredients just until combined.

5. Add the blueberries and stir.

6. Use cooking spray or butter to grease a muffin pan. Add batter to each muffin cup until it is 3/4 filled.

7. Bake for 20 to 25 minutes in a preheated oven, or until a toothpick inserted in the center of a muffin emerges clean.

8. Let the muffins cool for a few minutes in the muffin tin, then transfer them to a wire rack to cool completely.

Banana Bread

Ingredients:

- 1 1/2 cups of All-purpose flour
- 1 tsp of Baking powder
- 1/2 tsp of Salt
- 1/2 tsp of White sugar
- 2 Eggs
- 1/4 cup of Milk
- 1/4 cup of Vegetable oil
- 3 ripe, mashed Bananas

Method of Preparation:

1. Preheat the oven to 350°F.

2. Combine the flour, baking powder, salt, and sugar in a sizable mixing bowl. Mix thoroughly.

3. Beat the eggs in a separate bowl. Mix well after adding the milk and vegetable oil.

4. Combine the wet ingredients with the mashed bananas.

5. Combine the dry ingredients just before adding the wet ingredients.

6. Grease a loaf pan with butter or cooking spray. Pour the batter into the pan.

7. Bake in the preheated oven for 50-60 minutes, or until a toothpick inserted into the center of the bread comes out clean.

8. Let the bread cool for a few minutes in the pan, then transfer it to a wire rack to cool completely.

These muffins and breads are perfect for breakfast on the go or for a leisurely weekend brunch. They can be made ahead of time and stored in an airtight container, making them a convenient and delicious option for busy mornings. The blueberry muffins offer a burst of fruity flavor, while the banana bread provides a comforting and hearty taste. So why not give them a try and enjoy a satisfying breakfast?

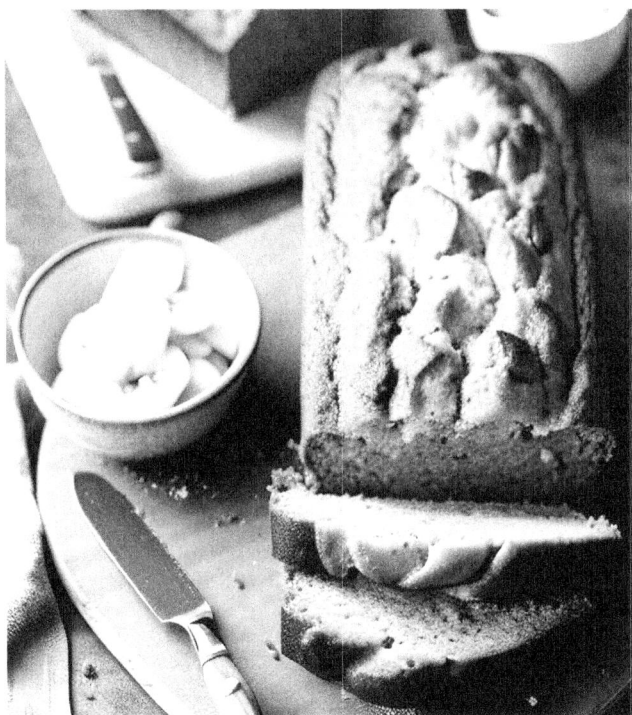

Banana Bread

CHAPTER FOUR

Snack Recipes

Quick And Easy Snacks For Weight Gain

Snacking can be a great way to boost your calorie intake throughout the day, especially if you're looking to gain weight. However, it can be difficult to find healthy snack options that are quick and easy to prepare. In this writing, we will explore some simple yet delicious snack recipes that can help you reach your weight gain goals.

Peanut Butter and Banana Toast

Ingredients:

- 2 Slices of Whole grain bread
- 2 tbsp of Peanut butter
- 1 Sliced Banana

Method of Preparation:

1. Toast the bread slices.

2. Spread the peanut butter evenly on each slice.

3. Top with sliced banana.

4. Serve immediately.

Avocado and Egg Toast

Ingredients:

•2 Slices of Whole grain bread
•1 mashed Avocado
•2 scrambled Eggs

Method of Preparation:

1. Toast the bread slices.

2. Spread the mashed avocado evenly on each slice.

3. Top with scrambled eggs.

4. Serve immediately.

Yogurt and Granola Parfait

Ingredients:

1 cup of Greek yogurt
1/2 cup of Granola
1/2 cup, fresh or frozen Berries

Method of Preparation:

1. In a small bowl, mix together the Greek yogurt and granola.

2. In a separate bowl, defrost the berries if using frozen.

3. Layer the yogurt and granola mixture with the berries in a serving glass or bowl.

4. Serve immediately.

These snacks are not only quick and easy to prepare, but they also offer a balance of protein, healthy fats, and carbohydrates to keep you satisfied and energized throughout the day. The peanut butter and banana toast provides a sweet and satisfying flavor, while the avocado and egg toast offers a savory and creamy taste. The yogurt and granola parfait offers a refreshing and crunchy texture with the added sweetness from the berries. You can also customize these snacks by adding different toppings or swapping out ingredients to suit your taste preferences.

Homemade Protein Bars And Energy Balls

Making your own protein bars and energy balls can be a wonderful option if you're searching for a quick, healthy snack to help your weight gain objectives. They can be tailored to your taste preferences and are simple to produce. Moreover, they are a fantastic source of protein and good fats, which can keep you pleased and full in between meals. We'll provide two scrumptious and wholesome protein bar and energy ball recipes in this writing.

Homemade Protein Bars

Ingredients:

- 1 Cup of Rolled oats
- 1/2 cup of Almond butter
- 1/2 cup of Honey
- 1 tsp of Vanilla extract
- 1/2 cup of Protein powder
- 1/2 cup of Dark chocolate chips

Method of Preparation:

1. In a large mixing bowl, combine the rolled oats, almond butter, honey, and vanilla extract. Mix well.

2. Add the protein powder and mix until everything is well combined.

3. Fold in the dark chocolate chips.

4. Line a baking dish with parchment paper.

5. Pour the mixture into the baking dish and press down firmly to make an even layer.

6. Place the baking dish in the refrigerator for at least 1 hour to set.

7. Cut into bars and store in an airtight container in the refrigerator.

Homemade Energy Balls

Ingredients:

• 1 cup, pitted of Medjool dates
• 1 Cup of Rolled oats
• 1/2 cup of Almond butter
• 1/4 cup of Chia seeds
• 1/4 cup of Honey
• 1/2 cup of Unsweetened shredded coconut

Method of Preparation:

1. In a food processor, blend the Medjool dates until they form a paste.

2. Add the rolled oats, almond butter, chia seeds, and honey to the food processor. Blend until everything is well combined.

3. Form the mixture into small balls.

4. Roll the balls in the unsweetened shredded coconut until they are coated.

5. Place the energy balls in the refrigerator for at least 30 minutes to set.

6.Keep chilled and in an airtight container.

These homemade protein bars and energy balls can be a great snack option for when you're on the go or need a quick boost of energy. They are easy to make and can be customized to your liking. Plus, they are a healthy and delicious way to support your weight gain goals.

Dips And Spreads With Crackers And Vegetables

Dips and spreads with crackers and vegetables are a delicious and nutritious snack option that can be enjoyed any time of day. Whether you're looking for a quick and easy snack to enjoy at work or a tasty appetizer to serve at a party, these dips and spreads are sure to satisfy. In this writing, we will share two tasty and simple recipes for dips and spreads that can be paired with crackers and vegetables.

Hummus Dip

Ingredients:

- 1 can, drained and rinsed of Chickpeas
- 1/4 cup of Tahini
- 2 cloves of Garlic

•2 tbsp of Lemon juice
•1 tbsp of Olive oil
•1/4 tsp of Salt
•1/4 cup of Paprika

Method of Preparation:

1. In a food processor, blend the chickpeas, tahini, garlic, lemon juice, and olive oil until smooth.

2. Add salt and paprika to the mixture and blend again.

3. If the mixture is too thick, add water 1 tbsp at a time until it reaches the desired consistency.

4. Transfer the hummus to a serving bowl and drizzle with olive oil and paprika.

5. Serve with crackers and vegetables.

Spinach and Artichoke Dip

Ingredients:

•Cream cheese: 8 oz, softened
•1/2 cup of Sour cream
•1/2 cup of Mayonnaise
•2 cloves, minced Garlic
•1 cup, cooked and chopped Spinach
•1 can, drained and chopped   Artichoke hearts
•1/2 cup, shredded Parmesan cheese
•1/4 tsp of Salt
•1/4 cup of Black pepper

Method of Preparation:

1. Preheat the oven to 375°F.

2. In a mixing bowl, combine the cream cheese, sour cream, mayonnaise, and garlic. Mix well.

3. Add the spinach, artichoke hearts, Parmesan cheese, salt, and black pepper to the mixture. Mix well.

4. Place the mixture in a baking dish that can go in the oven.

5. Bake in the preheated oven for 20-25 minutes, or until the top is golden brown and the dip is heated through.

6. Serve with crackers and vegetables.

Popcorn Variations

People of all ages like the common snack of popcorn. In addition to being delicious, it also makes a nutritious snack, especially when prepared without using excessive amounts of salt or butter. We'll discuss some delectable and simple popcorn varieties in this writing that are excellent for weight gainers. These quick and easy dishes can be made in a short amount of time.

Caramel Popcorn

Ingredients:

- 1/2 cup of Popcorn kernels
- 1/2 cup of Brown sugar
- 1/4 cup of Butter
- 1/4 cup of Corn syrup
- 1/4 tsp of Salt
- 1/4 cup of Baking soda

Method of Preparation:

1. Preheat the oven to 250°F.

2. Pop the popcorn kernels according to the package instructions and set aside.

3. In a saucepan, combine the brown sugar, butter, corn syrup, and salt. Boil the mixture until it boils while stirring continuously over medium heat.

4. After taking it off the heat, stir in the baking soda.

5. After drizzling the popcorn with the caramel mixture, toss it to coat.

6. Place the popcorn on a baking sheet covered with parchment paper, spread it out, and bake it for 30 minutes while stirring it every ten minutes.

7. Take the dish out of the oven, then let it cool before serving.

Spicy Popcorn

Ingredients:

• 1/2 cup of Popcorn kernels
• 2 tbsp of Butter
• 1 tsp of Chili powder
• 1 tsp of Cumin powder
• 1 tsp of Paprika
• 1/2 tsp of Garlic powder
• 1/4 tsp of Salt

Method of Preparation:

1. Pop the popcorn kernels according to the package instructions and set aside.

2. In a small bowl, mix together the chili powder, cumin powder, paprika, garlic powder, and salt.

3. Put the butter in a pot and heat it gently.

4. Add the spice mixture to the melted butter and stir to combine.

5. Pour the butter mixture over the popcorn and toss to coat.

6. Serve immediately.

Sweet and Salty Popcorn

Ingredients:

• 1/2 cup of Popcorn kernels

•2 tbsp of Butter
•2 tbsp of Brown sugar
•1/4 tsp of Salt

Method of Preparation:

1. Pop the popcorn kernels according to the package instructions and set aside.

2. Put the butter in a pan and heat it gently.
3. Add the brown sugar and salt to the melted butter and stir to combine.

4. Pour the butter mixture over the popcorn and toss to coat.

5. Serve immediately.

These popcorn variations are a great way to add some variety to your snacking routine. They are perfect for those who want to gain weight, as they are high in calories and can be made to suit individual taste preferences. So next time you're in the mood for a quick and easy snack, try making one of these delicious popcorn variations and enjoy.

Trail Mix And Granola Bars

Trail mix and granola bars are popular snacks that are perfect for those who want to gain weight. They are easy to prepare, portable, and can be customized to suit individual taste preferences. In this writing, I will share some delicious trail mix and granola bar recipes that are high in calories and packed with nutrients.

Trail Mix

Ingredients:

• 1 cup of Almonds
• 1 cup of Cashews
• 1 cup of Walnuts
• 1 cup of Dried cranberries
• 1 cup of Dark chocolate chips

Method of Preparation:

1. Preheat the oven to 350°F.

2. Spread the almonds, cashews, and walnuts on a baking sheet lined with parchment paper.

3. Roast the nuts in the oven for 10-15 minutes, or until golden brown and fragrant.

4. Allow the nuts to cool, then mix in the dried cranberries and dark chocolate chips.
5. Store the trail mix in an airtight container.

Granola Bars

Ingredients:

•2 cups of Rolled oats
•1 cup of Almonds
•1 cup of Walnuts
•1 cup of Dried cranberries
•1/2 cup of Honey
•1/4 cup of Brown sugar
•1/4 cup of Coconut oil
•1/4 tsp of Salt

Method of Preparation:

1. Preheat the oven to 350°F.

2. Spread the rolled oats, almonds, and walnuts on a baking sheet lined with parchment paper.

3. Roast the oats and nuts in the oven for 10-15 minutes, or until golden brown and fragrant.

4. In a saucepan, combine the honey, brown sugar, coconut oil, and salt. Boil the mixture until it boils while stirring continuously over medium heat.

5. Turn off the heat and stir in the dried cranberries, almonds, and walnuts that have been roasted.

6. Press the mixture into a 9x13-inch baking dish that has been greased.

7. Bake for 20 to 25 minutes, or until the top is golden.

8. Allow the granola bars to cool before cutting into squares.

These trail mix and granola bar recipes are a great way to satisfy your snack cravings while also providing your body with the nutrients it needs to support weight gain. They are easy to prepare, can be customized to suit individual taste preferences, and are perfect for on-the-go snacking.

Cheese And Fruit Plates

Cheese and fruit plates make for a delicious and nutritious snack that can help with weight gain. Not only are they a great source of protein and healthy fats, but they're also loaded with vitamins and minerals from the variety of fruits used. In this recipe, we'll be using a selection of cheeses and fruits to create a plate that's not only satisfying but also visually appealing.

Ingredients:

- 1 cup of sliced cheddar cheese
- 1 cup of sliced gouda cheese
- 1 cup of sliced brie cheese
- 2 cups of sliced grapes
- 2 cups of sliced strawberries
- 2 cups of sliced kiwi
- 1 cup of sliced pineapple
- 1 cup of sliced apples
- 1 cup of sliced pears
- 1/2 cup of mixed nuts

Method of Preparation:

1. Start by arranging the sliced cheeses on a large plate or platter. You can arrange them in a circle or create a more creative design by overlapping them in different ways.

2. Next, add the sliced fruits around the cheese. You can choose to group similar fruits together or mix and match them for a more visually appealing presentation.

2. Sprinkle the mixed nuts on top of the cheese and fruit platter for some added crunch and texture.

4. Serve the cheese and fruit plate as is or with some crackers or bread on the side for an extra filling snack.

Tips:

• Be sure to choose a variety of cheeses with different textures and flavors for a more dynamic plate.

• Use fresh and in-season fruits for the best taste and texture.

• If you're not a fan of nuts, you can omit them or substitute them with seeds or dried fruits instead.

• To make the plate even more filling, add some slices of cured meat or salami alongside the cheese and fruit.

Smoothie Bowls

Smoothie bowls have become a popular snack choice for many health-conscious individuals. They're packed with nutrients, easy to make, and can be customized to suit individual tastes and preferences. In this recipe, we'll be using a variety of fruits and other ingredients to create a delicious and filling smoothie bowl that's perfect for a mid-day snack.

Ingredients:

•1 cup of frozen mixed berries (strawberries, blueberries, raspberries)
•1 banana
•1 cup of almond milk
•1 tbsp of chia seeds
•1 tbsp of honey
•1/4 cup of granola
•1/4 cup of sliced fresh fruit (kiwi, mango, or any other fruit of your choice)

Method of Preparation:

1. First, blend the frozen mixed berries, almond milk, banana, chia seeds, and honey in a food processor or blender until smooth. More almond milk can be added if the mixture is too thick.

2. Place the bowl with the blended mixture in it.

3. Add the granola and fresh fruit slices to the smoothie bowl as a garnish.

4. Serve and consume right away.

Tips:

• In place of almond milk, you can use any type of milk you like, including cow's milk, soy milk, or oat milk.

• Flaxseeds or hemp seeds can be used as a substitute for chia seeds if you don't have any on hand.

• Before combining the smoothie ingredients, you can add a scoop of protein powder for more protein.

• Add your preferred toppings, such as almonds, coconut flakes, or chocolate chips, to create a unique smoothie bowl.

• Depending on the fruit you have on hand, use fresh or frozen fruit.

• You can blend the smoothie mixture with less liquid if you desire a thicker consistency.

If you're feeling tired of spending long hours in the kitchen, I have the perfect option for you: "A smoothie recipe book".

With quick and easy-to-prepare recipes that are packed with nutrients and calories, you can get all the benefits of a healthy smoothie without the fuss while achieving your weight gain goals. Whether you're looking for a delicious breakfast, post-workout snack, or a refreshing treat, this smoothie recipe book for weight gain has got you covered. So why not check it out and see how easy and enjoyable healthy eating can be?

CLICK HERE TO GET SMOOTHIE RECIPES FOR WEIGHT GAIN

Yoghurt Bowls

Yoghurt bowls are a tasty and nutritious snack that can be enjoyed any time of day. They're easy to make and can be customized with a variety of toppings to suit individual tastes and preferences. In this recipe, we'll be using Greek yoghurt as the base and adding a variety of fruits, nuts, and other ingredients for a delicious and satisfying snack.

Ingredients:

• 1 cup of Greek yoghurt
• 1/4 cup of mixed nuts (almonds, walnuts, cashews)

• 1/4 cup of mixed fresh fruit (berries, kiwi, mango)
• 1 tbsp of honey
• 1 tbsp of chia seeds
• 1/4 cup of granola

Method of Preparation:

1. Pour the Greek yogurt into a bowl first.

2. Top the yoghurt with the mixed nuts and fresh fruit.

3. Drizzle the fruit and nuts with the honey.

4. Top the yoghurt bowl with the chia seeds and granola.

5. Serve and consume right away.

Tips:

• You can use any variety of yoghurt, including ordinary, low-fat, and fat-free varieties.

- Add your preferred toppings, such as shredded coconut, sliced bananas, or chocolate chips, to personalize your yoghurt bowl.

- Depending on the fruit you have on hand, use fresh or frozen fruit.

- You can use flaxseeds or hemp seeds in place of chia seeds if you don't like them.

- Before putting the toppings over the yoghurt, you can add a scoop of protein powder for more protein.

- You can increase the amount of honey or use maple syrup or agave nectar in place of honey if you prefer a sweeter flavor.

Toast And Sandwich Variations

A quick and simple snack choice that can be tailored to individual tastes and preferences is various toast and sandwich options. While they may be cooked with nutrient-dense ingredients, they can also be a fantastic alternative for anyone trying to gain weight. This recipe will show you how to make three different toast and sandwich versions that are ideal for a mid-afternoon snack utilizing a variety of ingredients.

Variation 1: Avocado Toast

Ingredients:

- 2 slices of whole grain bread
- 1 ripe avocado
- 1 tbsp of olive oil
- 1/4 tsp of salt
- 1/4 tsp of black pepper
- Optional toppings: sliced tomato, sliced cucumber, crumbled feta cheese

Method of Preparation:

1. To begin, toast the bread slices in a toaster or toaster oven until they are just lightly browned.

2. Halve the avocado and scoop out the pit while the bread is toasting. To make the flesh smooth, scoop it out into a basin and mash it with a fork.

3. Add the salt, black pepper, and olive oil and mix thoroughly.

4. Top the toasted bread slices with the avocado mixture.

5. If desired, add any extra toppings.

6. Serve and consume right away.

Variation 2: Turkey and Cheese Sandwich

Ingredients:

•2 slices of whole grain bread
•3-4 slices of turkey breast
•1 slice of cheese (cheddar or Swiss)
•1 tbsp of mayonnaise
•1/4 tsp of black pepper

•Optional toppings: sliced tomato, sliced avocado, lettuce

Method of Preparation:

1. To begin, lightly brown the bread slices in a toaster or toaster oven.

2. Mayonnaise should be applied to one slice of bread.

3. Place a slice of cheese and a slice of turkey on the same piece of bread.

4. If desired, add any extra garnishes.

5. Add an additional slice of bread on top.

6. Present and devour right away.

Variation 3: Peanut Butter and Banana Toast

Ingredients:

•2 slices of whole grain bread
•2 tbsp of natural peanut butter
•1 banana, sliced
•Optional toppings: honey, sliced strawberries, chia seeds

Method of Preparation:

1. Initially, lightly brown the bread slices in a toaster or toaster oven.

2. The toasted bread slices are covered with peanut butter.

3. Place a banana slice on top.

4. If wished, include any extra garnishes.

5. If you'd like, drizzle with honey.

6. Serve right away and take pleasure in.
Tips:

•You are free to use any bread you like, including white, wheat, or sourdough.

• Opt for a natural peanut butter without extra sugars or oils.

• You can use any kind of cheese you like, including provolone, Swiss, or cheddar.

• Add your preferred toppings to your sandwiches, such as bacon, lettuce, or avocado slices.

• For the finest flavor, choose an avocado that is fully ripe and somewhat soft to the touch.

• For the peanut butter and banana toast variant, experiment with various nut butters and fruits.

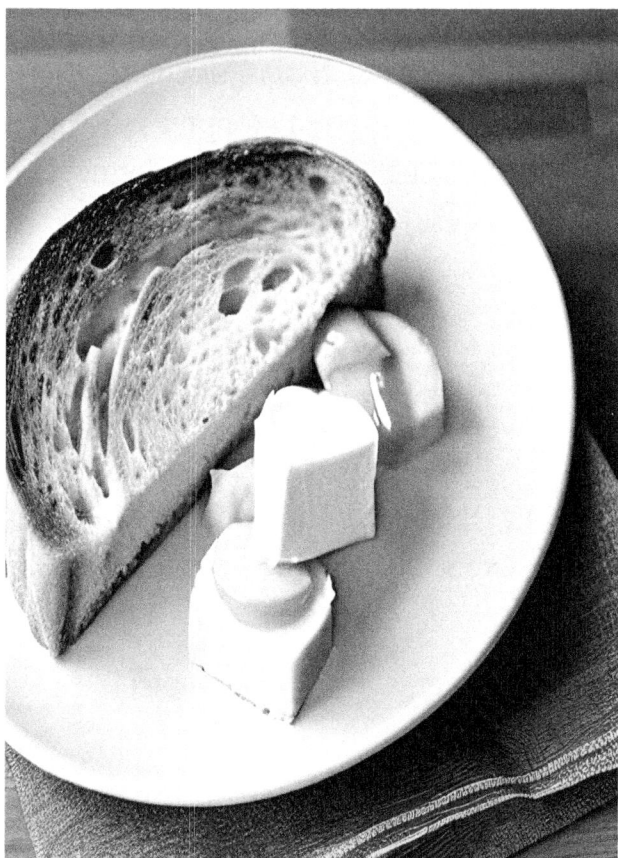

Peanut Butter And Banana Toast

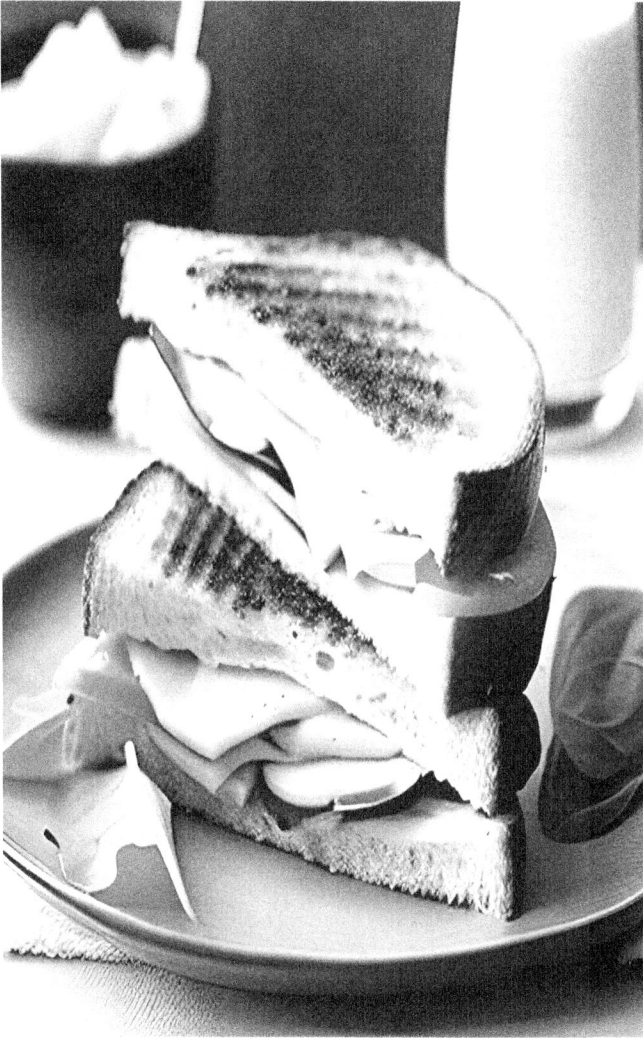

Turkey And Cheese Sandwich

CHAPTER FIVE

Lunch Recipes

Sandwiches And Wraps

Sandwiches and wraps are great choices for anyone trying to gain weight since they are simple to adapt to your dietary requirements. They may be cooked ahead of time and transported with you on the go, making them a convenient and delectable option for a noon meal.

You will need a few essential components to construct a filling sandwich or wrap that will aid in weight gain. Some of the ingredients you can use are listed below:

Ingredients:

•Bread or tortilla wraps
•Protein source (such as chicken, turkey, beef, tofu, or beans)

•Cheese
•Vegetables (such as lettuce, spinach, tomato, cucumber, and avocado)
•Condiments (such as mayonnaise, mustard, or hummus)

Method of Preparation:

1. Select your bread or tortilla wrap first. To add more nourishment, choose whole-grain bread or a tortilla wrap high in fiber.

2. Determine the protein source. Cook and slice your meat thinly if you're using chicken or beef. If you're using tofu, prepare it as directed on the package and cut it into little pieces. Beans should be drained, rinsed, and set aside if you're using them.

3. Cut your vegetables into bite-sized pieces or thin strips. Any type of vegetable will do, but be sure to add a few leafy greens for extra nourishment.

4. Select the cheese. Any sort of cheese is acceptable, but a mild cheese, such as Swiss or cheddar, will work best in a sandwich or wrap.

5. Select your dipping sauces. You can add any condiment you like, including hummus, mustard, and mayonnaise.

6. Place your tortilla or bread wrap flat on a tidy surface. Put your preferred condiment on the tortilla or bread.

7. Top the condiment with your protein source. Make careful to stack chicken or beef evenly if you're using either. Spread the tofu or beans you're using on the tortilla or bread equally.

8. Place your vegetables in a layer on top of the protein.To ensure that every bite contains a variety of vegetables, make sure you distribute them equally.

9. Cover the vegetables with your cheese.

10. Fold the sandwich in half or roll up the tortilla. When desired, divide the sandwich or wrap into halves or quarters.

11. Delight in your tasty and filling sandwich or wrap!

Salads With Protein And Healthy Fats

Salads are a great choice for people who want to have a healthy diet and get adequate protein and good fats. Having a well-balanced salad for lunch can provide you all the nutrients you need to feel satisfied and full. Here is a recipe for a salad that will satisfy your cravings and give you the energy you need to go through the rest of the day.

Ingredients:

•2 cups of mixed greens (spinach, lettuce, and arugula)
•1 cup of cooked quinoa
•1/2 cup of sliced cherry tomatoes
•1/2 cup of sliced cucumber

- 1/4 cup of sliced avocado
- 1/4 cup of sliced almonds
- 1/4 cup of crumbled feta cheese
- 4 oz of grilled chicken breast

Dressing:

- 2 tbsp of olive oil
- 1 tbsp of balsamic vinegar
- 1 tsp of Dijon mustard
- 1 tsp of honey
- Salt and pepper to taste

Method of Preparation:

1. First, prepare your quinoa by following the directions on the package. Place it aside to cool after cooking.

2. Heat an outdoor grill or grill pan to medium-high. Salt and pepper the chicken breast before grilling it for 6-7 minutes on each side, or until it is thoroughly done. Place it aside to cool after cooking.

3. Put your mixed greens in a sizable salad bowl after washing and drying them.

4. Slice the cucumbers and cherry tomatoes, then add them to the salad bowl.

5. Halve the avocado and scoop out the pit. Add the avocado to the salad dish after slicing it into thin pieces.

6. Combine all the ingredients in the salad bowl with the cooked quinoa.

7. Add the thinly sliced grilled chicken breast to the salad bowl.

8. Top the salad with the feta cheese crumbles and sliced almonds.

9. To prepare the dressing, mix together the olive oil, balsamic vinegar, honey, Dijon mustard, salt, and pepper in a small bowl.

10. Pour the dressing over the salad and toss to combine, coating the salad completely.

11. Present and savor your delectable and healthy salad!

For people trying to maintain a balanced diet while still ingesting enough nutrients to feel full and pleased, salads with protein and healthy fats are a great choice.by using high-quality ingredients and a well-balanced dressing, you can create a tasty and satisfying salad that will keep you feeling energized and focused throughout the day.

Vegetarian And Vegan Dishes

For individuals wishing to eat a plant-based diet or consume less meat and other animal products, vegetarian and vegan cuisine are a great choice. They are a fantastic alternative for lunch as well because they are simple to make ahead of time and transport. Here is a recipe for a tasty, wholesome vegetarian or vegan supper that will sate both your appetite and your palate.

Ingredients:

- 1 cup of quinoa
- 1 can of black beans
- 1 red bell pepper, diced
- 1/2 red onion, diced
- 1/2 cup of frozen corn
- 1 avocado, diced
- 1 lime, juiced
- 2 tbsp of chopped cilantro
- Salt and pepper to taste

Method of Preparation:

1. First, prepare your quinoa by following the directions on the package. Place it aside to cool after cooking.

1. Drain, rinse, and set aside the black beans.

3. Cut the red onion and bell pepper into dice and place them aside.

4. Heat the frozen corn completely in a small saucepan over medium heat.

Place it aside to cool after cooking.

5. Combine the cooked quinoa, cooled corn, diced red onion, diced red bell pepper, and diced black beans in a big bowl.

6. Combine the diced avocado, lime juice, cilantro, salt, and pepper in a different bowl. To evenly coat the avocado, combine all the ingredients in a mixing bowl.

7. Fill the bowl with the quinoa and black bean mixture and add the avocado mixture to it.

8. Combine everything until the black bean and quinoa mixture is thoroughly mixed with the avocado mixture.

9. Dish up your scrumptious and wholesome vegetarian or vegan dish and enjoy!

Pasta and Noodles Dishes

Spaghetti and noodles meals are a popular option for lunch and can be an ideal alternative for individuals seeking to gain weight.

You may make a tasty and nutritious meal that will help you achieve your weight gain objectives by combining protein and healthy fats in the right proportions with high-quality products. Here is a recipe for a satisfying and substantial pasta dish that will give you energy and a sensation of fullness.

Ingredients:

•8 oz of whole wheat pasta
•1 tbsp of olive oil
•1 onion, diced
•3 cloves of garlic, minced
•1 can of diced tomatoes
•1/2 cup of vegetable broth
•1/2 cup of chopped fresh basil
•1/4 cup of chopped fresh parsley
•1/4 cup of grated parmesan cheese
•Salt and pepper to taste

Method of Preparation:

1. Start by cooking your pasta as directed on the package.
Place it aside to cool after cooking.

2. In a big skillet over medium heat, warm the olive oil while the pasta is cooking.

3. Add the diced onion to the skillet and cook for 5 to 7 minutes, or until translucent and soft.

4. After adding the minced garlic to the skillet, cook it for an additional one to two minutes, or until it begins to smell good.

5. Stir in the vegetable broth and diced tomatoes before bringing the mixture to a simmer.

6. Stir in the freshly chopped parsley and basil, and let the mixture simmer for 5-7 minutes, or until it slightly thickens.

7. Include the cooked pasta and toss everything in the skillet to evenly distribute the tomato sauce over the pasta.

8. Top the pasta with the grated parmesan cheese and combine everything once more.

9. To taste, add salt and pepper to the pasta.

10. Present and savor your filling and delicious pasta dish!

Rice And Grain Dishes

Several cuisines around the world use rice and grain dishes as a main ingredient, and they may make a tasty and wholesome lunch. You may make a nutritious and fulfilling dinner that will keep you energized all day by combining whole grains, vegetables, and protein. This is a recipe for a delightful, nutritious rice and grain meal that you can make in just a few minutes and is great for lunch.

Ingredients:

- 1 cup of brown rice
- 1 cup of quinoa
- 1 can of chickpeas
- 1 red bell pepper, diced
- 1/2 red onion, diced
- 1/2 cup of frozen peas
- 1/4 cup of chopped fresh parsley
- 1/4 cup of chopped fresh mint
- 2 tbsp of olive oil
- 1 lemon, juiced
- Salt and pepper to taste

Method of Preparation:

1. Start by preparing your brown rice and quinoa in accordance with the directions on the package. Place them aside to cool after cooking.

2. Drain and rinse the chickpeas in the can, then reserve them.

3. Cut the red onion and bell pepper into dice and place them aside.

4. Heat the frozen peas in a small saucepan over medium heat until they are thoroughly heated. Place them aside to cool after cooking.

5. Combine the cooked quinoa, chickpeas, diced red onion, diced red bell pepper, and cooled peas in a big bowl.

6. In a different bowl, mix the lemon juice and olive oil. Add salt and pepper to the food according to taste.

7. After adding the dressing, combine the rice and grain mixture and stir it all together until the dressing is distributed evenly.

8. Recommend adding the mint and freshly chopped parsley to the bowl and mixing everything once more.

9. Dish up your delicious and nutritious rice and grain dish and savor it!

Soups And Broths

Soups and broths are a great option for a healthy and filling lunch. They can provide a variety of nutrients while also being low in calories, making them an ideal choice for those looking to gain weight. Here is a recipe for a delicious and hearty soup that is perfect for lunch and will help you reach your weight gain goals.

Ingredients:

• 1 onion, diced
• 2 cloves of garlic, minced
• 2 carrots, peeled and diced
• 2 celery stalks, diced
• 1 red bell pepper, diced
• 4 cups of chicken or vegetable broth
• 1 can of diced tomatoes
• 1 can of chickpeas
• 1/2 cup of quinoa
• 1 tsp of dried oregano

•1 tsp of dried basil
•Salt and pepper to taste
•1 tbsp of olive oil

Method of Preparation:

1. To start, warm up the olive oil in a sizable pot over medium heat.

2. Stir in the diced onion and cook, stirring occasionally, for 5 to 7 minutes, or until the onion is soft and translucent.

3. Include the minced garlic in the pot and cook for an additional one to two minutes, or until the garlic is fragrant.

4. Add the diced carrots, celery, and red bell pepper to the pot and simmer for 5-7 minutes, or until the vegetables have softened.

5. Include the broth, diced tomatoes, and can of chickpeas in the mixture and bring it to a simmer.

6. Stir in the quinoa and simmer the soup for 20 to 25 minutes, or until the quinoa is cooked and the vegetables are soft.

7. To taste, add salt and pepper to the soup.

8. Dish up your hearty and delicious soup and savor it!

Dinner Recipes

High-protein, High-Calorie Meals

It's crucial to eat meals heavy in protein and calories if you want to gain weight. By doing this, you can make sure that your body is receiving the nutrients and energy it needs to add muscle and gain weight. Here is a recipe for a high-protein, high-calorie dinner that is delicious, satisfying, and ideal for people trying to gain weight.

Ingredients:

•1 pound of ground beef or turkey

- 1 can of black beans, drained and rinsed
- 1 red bell pepper, diced
- 1 green bell pepper, diced
- 1 onion, diced
- 2 cloves of garlic, minced
- 1 can of diced tomatoes
- 1/2 cup of quinoa
- 1 cup of chicken or vegetable broth
- 1 tsp of chili powder
- 1 tsp of cumin
- Salt and pepper to taste
- Shredded cheddar cheese for topping

Method of Preparation:

1. Start by browning the ground beef or turkey over medium heat in a big skillet. Cook until crumbled and browned.

2. Add the minced garlic, onion, and diced red and green bell peppers to the skillet with the ground beef. The vegetables should be sautéed for 5-7 minutes, or until they are soft.

3. Add quinoa, chicken or vegetable broth, cumin, chili powder, and a rinsed and drained can of diced tomatoes to the skillet. Mix all of the ingredients.

4. After bringing the mixture to a boil, reduce the heat to a simmer, cover the pan, and cook the quinoa for 20 to 25 minutes, or until it is tender and the liquid has thickened.

5. Add salt and pepper to taste and season the mixture.

6. Once the mixture is cooked, top it with shredded cheddar cheese and allow it to melt.

7. Serve and enjoy your delicious high-protein, high-calorie meal

Easy-To-Make One-Pot Dishes

For hectic weeknights when you don't have the time or energy to make a complicated meal, one-pot meals are a lifesaver.

These meals are the ideal choice for anyone who wants to have a great and healthy dinner without spending hours in the kitchen because they are simple to prepare and require little cleanup.

You can try one of the simple one-pot meals listed below for dinner:

One-Pot Tomato Basil Pasta

Ingredients:

- 1 pound spaghetti
- 1 can of diced tomatoes
- 4 cups of vegetable broth
- 1 onion, chopped
- 4 cloves of garlic, minced
- 2 tablespoons of olive oil
- 1 teaspoon of salt
- 1 teaspoon of black pepper
- 1/4 cup of fresh basil, chopped

Method of Preparation:

1. Saute the onion and garlic in the olive oil

in a large pot until fragrant and translucent.

2. Fill the pot with the spaghetti, diced tomatoes, vegetable broth, salt, and pepper.

3. Increase the heat to a boil, then lower it to a simmer.

4. Until the spaghetti is tender and the liquid has been absorbed, cook for 12 to 15 minutes.

5. Add the basil that has been chopped and mix well.

6. Present hot and savor

One-Pot Chicken and Rice

Ingredients:

•4 chicken thighs
•1 cup of white rice
•1 onion, chopped
•4 cloves of garlic, minced

•2 cups of chicken broth
• 1 can of diced tomatoes
• 1 teaspoon of salt
• 1 teaspoon of black pepper
•2 tablespoons of olive oil

Method of Preparation:

1. Set the oven's temperature to 375°F (190°C).

2. Heat the olive oil in a sizable oven-safe pot over medium-high heat.

3. Brown the chicken thighs on both sides in a hot skillet.

4. Take out the chicken and set it aside.

5. Saute the onion and garlic in the same pot until they are fragrant and translucent.

6. Add the diced tomatoes, salt, and black pepper to the pot along with the white rice and stir to combine.

7. Top the rice mixture with the chicken thighs.

8. Place the pot in the preheated oven, cover it with a lid, and bake for 35 to 40 minutes, or until the rice is tender and the chicken is thoroughly cooked.

9. Take it out of the oven and give it a five to ten minute rest before serving.

One-Pot Veggie Chili

Ingredients:

- 1 can of rinsed and drained black beans
- 1 can of kidney beans, drained and rinsed
- 1 can of diced tomatoes
- 2 cups of vegetable broth
- 1 onion, chopped
- 4 cloves of garlic, minced
- 1 bell pepper, chopped
- 1 zucchini, chopped
- 1 teaspoon of chili powder
- 1 teaspoon of cumin

•1 teaspoon of salt
•1 teaspoon of black pepper
•2 tablespoons of olive oil

Method of Preparation:

1. Heat the olive oil in a big pot over a medium-high heat.

2. Sauté the zucchini, bell pepper, onion, and garlic until they are tender and fragrant.

3. Stir in the black beans, kidney beans, diced tomatoes, vegetable broth, cumin, chili powder, salt, and black pepper.

4. After the mixture comes to a boil, lower the heat to a simmer.

5. Sauté the vegetables for 20 to 25 minutes, or until they are soft.

Meat and Poultry Dishes

Meat and poultry meals might be a great addition to your diet if you're trying to gain weight. They are also loaded with important nutrients like iron and zinc. Their high protein content can aid in the development of lean muscle mass.

The following dishes for meat and poultry dinners are excellent for gaining weight:

Beef Stroganoff

Ingredients:

- 1 pound of beef sirloin, thinly sliced
- 1 onion, chopped
- 4 cloves of garlic, minced
- 1 cup of beef broth
- 1 cup of sour cream
- 2 tablespoons of butter
- 2 tablespoons of flour
- Salt and pepper to taste
- 8 ounces of egg noodles, cooked

Method of Preparation:

1. Melt the butter in a sizable pan over medium-high heat.

2. Include the beef and cook it until it is evenly browned.

3. Take the beef out of the skillet and place it aside.

4. Saute the onion and garlic in the same pan until they are fragrant and soft.

5. Stir the flour into the mixture in the pan.

6. Continuously stir in the beef broth while adding it gradually.

7. Include the sour cream in the pan and stir to combine.

8. Return the beef to the pan and give it a quick stir to coat it with the sauce.

9. Taste the meal and season with salt and pepper.

10. Put the cooked egg noodles on top of the stroganoff.

Lemon and Herb Roasted Chicken

Ingredients:

- 1 whole chicken, cleaned and patted dry
- 2 lemons, sliced
- 1/4 cup of olive oil
- 1 tablespoon of dried oregano
- 1 tablespoon of dried thyme
- Salt and pepper to taste

Method of Preparation:

1. Set your oven to 375°F (190°C) before using it.

2. Combine the oregano, thyme, olive oil, salt, and pepper in a small bowl.

3. Apply the mixture to the chicken by rubbing it all over, being sure to get inside the cavity and beneath the skin.

4. Place the sliced lemons inside the cavity.

5. Put the chicken in a roasting pan and roast it in the preheated oven for 1 to 1.5 hours, or until it reaches a temperature of 165°F (74°C) inside.

6. Before carving and serving, let the chicken rest for 10-15 minutes.

Spicy Beef Stir-Fry

Ingredients:

•1 pound of beef sirloin, thinly sliced
•1 onion, chopped
•1 bell pepper, sliced
•2 cups of broccoli florets
•4 cloves of garlic, minced
•2 tablespoons of vegetable oil
•2 tablespoons of soy sauce
•1 tablespoon of honey
•1 teaspoon of sriracha sauce
•Salt and pepper to taste

Method of Preparation:

1. Heat the vegetable oil over high heat in a sizable wok or pan.

2. Include the beef and stir-fry it until it is evenly browned.

3. Take the beef out of the skillet and place it aside.

4. Sauté the onion, bell pepper, broccoli, and garlic in the same pan until they are soft and fragrant.

5. Combine the soy sauce, honey, and sriracha sauce in a small bowl.

6. After adding the sauce to the pan of vegetables, stir them together.

7. Return the beef to the pan and give it a quick stir to coat it with the sauce.

8. To taste, add salt and pepper to the dish.

9. Arrange rice or noodles on top of the stir-fry.

Seafood Dishes

It's good news if you enjoy seafood. In addition to being delicious, seafood dishes are also a great source of protein, Omega-3 fatty acids, and a number of vitamins and minerals. The following dishes for seafood dinners are sure to please:

Garlic Butter Shrimp

Ingredients:

•1 pound of shrimp, peeled and deveined
•4 cloves of garlic, minced
•1/2 cup of butter
•1/4 cup of fresh parsley, chopped
•1/4 teaspoon of red pepper flakes
•Salt and pepper to taste

Method of Preparation:

1. Heat the butter to a medium-high temperature in a sizable pan.

2. Add the garlic to the pan and cook it along with the red pepper flakes until the garlic is fragrant.

3. Add the shrimp to the pan, and cook them for about 2-3 minutes per side, or until they are pink and cooked through.

4. Add pepper and salt to taste before spicing the shrimp.

5. Just before serving, garnish with parsley.

Lemon Garlic Salmon

Ingredients:

•4 salmon fillets
•4 cloves of garlic, minced
•1/4 cup of olive oil

•1/4 cup of fresh lemon juice
•1/4 cup of fresh parsley, chopped
•Salt and pepper to taste

Method of Preparation:

1. Preheat your oven to 375°F (190°C).

2. In a small bowl, mix together the garlic, olive oil, lemon juice, parsley, salt, and pepper.

3. Place the salmon fillets on a baking sheet and spoon the garlic and lemon mixture over the top.

4. Bake in the preheated oven for 12-15 minutes, or until the salmon is cooked through.

5. Garnish with additional chopped parsley before serving.

Seafood Paella

Ingredients:

- 1 pound of shrimp, peeled and deveined
- 1 pound of mussels, cleaned and debearded
- 1 pound of clams, cleaned
- 1/2 pound of chorizo sausage, sliced
- 1 onion, chopped
- 4 cloves of garlic, minced
- 1 red bell pepper, chopped
- 1/4 cup of olive oil
- 2 cups of Arborio rice
- 4 cups of chicken broth
- 1 teaspoon of smoked paprika
- Salt and pepper to taste

Method of Preparation:

1. Heat the olive oil in a sizable paella pan or skillet over medium-high heat.

2. Place the chorizo sausage in the pan and cook it until it is evenly browned.

3. Take the sausage out of the pan and place it to the side.

4. In the same pan, sauté the onion, garlic, and red bell pepper until they become tender and fragrant.

5. Add the Arborio rice to the pan and stir to coat it in the oil and vegetables.

6. Pour in the chicken broth and add the smoked paprika.

7. Bring the mixture to a simmer and let it cook for 10-15 minutes, or until the rice is almost cooked through.

8. Add the shrimp, mussels, clams, and chorizo sausage to the pan and stir to combine.

9. Cover the pan and let the seafood cook for 5-7 minutes, or until the shrimp are pink and the mussels and clams have opened.

10. Spice up with salt and pepper to taste before serving.

These seafood dinner recipes are perfect for any occasion, from a casual weeknight meal to a special dinner party. They're delicious, healthy, and easy to make, so why not give them a try?

Stews and Chilis

Traditional comfort foods like stews and chili are ideal for chilly winter nights. They can be a wonderful addition to a diet plan for weight gain in addition to being delicious and filling. You may prepare a delightful and satisfying dinner that will assist you in reaching your calorie objectives by utilizing high-quality components and putting an emphasis on nutrient-dense foods.

ingredients:

•Protein:
Getting enough protein is one of the most crucial elements of a diet for weight gain.

This macronutrient is crucial for weight gain because it helps to create and repair muscular tissue. Use lean ground beef, chicken breast, turkey, or a plant-based protein source like beans, lentils, or tofu to make a substantial stew or chili.

•Carbohydrates:
Carbohydrates are essential for weight gain since they give you energy for exercise and refill your muscles' glycogen stores. Choose complex sources of carbs like sweet potatoes, brown rice, or quinoa.

•Healthy Fats:
While it's necessary to keep your intake of trans and saturated fats to a minimum, healthy fats are a crucial component of any diet that targets weight gain. These fats aid in supplying vital nutrients and encouraging satiety, which can help you feel content and full for longer after meals. Avocado, olive oil, almonds, and seeds are a few excellent choices for healthy fats.

•Additional ingredients:
Add a variety of veggies like tomatoes, onions, and bell peppers to your stew or chili to boost taste and nutrition. Moreover, you can include herbs and spices like paprika, cumin, chili powder, and garlic powder.

Method of Preparation:

1. Start by heating a large pot over medium heat and adding a tablespoon of olive oil.

2. Add chopped onions and sauté until they are translucent, about 5 minutes.

3. Add chopped bell peppers and sauté for another 5 minutes.

4. Add your protein source, such as lean ground beef, and cook until browned.

5. Add canned tomatoes, diced sweet potatoes, and a cup of water. Bring to a boil and then reduce heat to a simmer.

6. Add your spices and herbs, such as chili powder, cumin, and garlic powder, and simmer for about 30 minutes.

7. Add a can of black beans and continue to simmer for another 10-15 minutes.

8. Taste and adjust seasoning as needed.

9. Serve hot with a side of brown rice or quinoa.

This hearty stew or chili is a delicious and filling dinner that can help you gain weight. The combination of protein, complex carbohydrates, and healthy fats will provide the nutrients you need to fuel your workouts and build muscle. Plus, the added fiber from the vegetables and beans will help keep you full and satisfied.

CHAPTER SIX

Sides And Accompaniments

Roasted Vegetables And Potatoes

Roasted vegetables and potatoes are a delicious and healthy side dish that can be served with a variety of main courses. This dish is easy to prepare and can be customized to your taste preferences by using different vegetables and seasonings. Here's a step-by-step guide to making roasted vegetables and potatoes:

Ingredients:

•Assorted vegetables such as carrots, broccoli, cauliflower, zucchini, bell peppers, and onions
•Potatoes
•Olive oil
•Salt
•Pepper

•Herbs of your choice (such as thyme, rosemary, or oregano)

Method of Preparation:

1. Set your oven to 400 fahrenheit.

2. Cut your vegetables into bite-sized pieces after washing them. Your potatoes should be peeled and cut into small pieces as well.

3. Arrange the diced potatoes and vegetables on a sizable baking sheet that has been lined with parchment paper.

4. Use just enough olive oil to lightly coat the potatoes and vegetables. When desired, season with salt and pepper.

5. Using your hands or a spatula, toss the potatoes and vegetables to distribute the seasoning and olive oil evenly.

6. Top the potatoes and vegetables with your chosen herbs.

7. Roast the baking sheet in the oven for 25 to 30 minutes, or until the potatoes and vegetables are fork-tender and well-browned.

8. After the vegetables and potatoes are done, take the baking sheet out of the oven and allow it to cool for a few minutes.

9. Accompany your main course with the roasted potatoes and vegetables.

This recipe is flexible and can be altered to your preferences. For added flavor, you could, for instance, add garlic or ginger to the vegetables. You could also add grated parmesan cheese to the potatoes and vegetables after they have been roasted to give them a cheesy touch. To give the dish a unique flavor, you may also experiment with using other herbs or spices.

Roasted vegetables and potatoes are a healthy and delicious side dish that pairs well with a variety of main courses. This recipe is easy to prepare and can be customized to your liking, making it a great addition to your dinner repertoire.

Grilled Fruits And Vegetables

Grilled fruits and vegetables are a healthy and delicious side dish that can be a great addition to a weight gain diet plan. Not only do they provide important nutrients and fiber, but they also add a burst of flavor to your meals. Here's a step-by-step guide to making grilled fruits and vegetables:

Ingredients:

•Assorted vegetables such as zucchini, bell peppers, onions, eggplant, and mushrooms
Assorted fruits such as pineapple, peaches, and mangoes
•Olive oil
•Salt
•Pepper
•Balsamic vinegar (optional)

Method of Preparation:

1. Set the grill to a medium-high temperature.

2. Cut your vegetables into big, bite-sized pieces after washing them.

3. Separate your fruits into pieces of similar sizes as well.

4. Combine olive oil, salt, and pepper in a small bowl. On the fruits and vegetables, brush the mixture.

5. Place the fruits and vegetables on the grill, turn them over occasionally, and cook for 10 to 15 minutes, or until they are soft and just charred.

6. Take the fruits and vegetables off the grill, and give them some time to cool.

7. Include the grilled fruits and vegetables as a side dish with your main course. Before

serving, sprinkle them with balsamic vinegar for an added flavor boost.

Fruits and vegetables that have been grilled are a flexible side dish that may be tailored to your preferences. To make a cuisine that appeals to your palate, you can experiment with various fruits and vegetables, as well as sauces and marinades. Consider adding some garlic or ginger to the mixture of olive oil for added flavor, or marinate the fruits and veggies in a marinade made of soy sauce for an Asian-inspired touch.

An excellent approach to increase the amount of nutrient-dense foods in your diet is by adding grilled fruits and vegetables to any meal.They are also a great option for weight gain, as they provide fiber, vitamins, and minerals, while also helping to fill you up and keep you satisfied. Give this recipe a try and enjoy a tasty and nutritious side dish that will leave you feeling satisfied and energized.

Baked Beans And Legumes

Baked beans and legumes are a classic side dish that are not only delicious, but also packed with protein and fiber, making them a great addition to a balanced diet. Here's a step-by-step guide to making baked beans and legumes:

Ingredients:

• 1 can of beans (such as navy, kidney, or black beans)
• 1 onion, diced
• 2 cloves of garlic, minced
• 1 tablespoon of olive oil
• 1/2 cup of tomato sauce
• 1/4 cup of molasses
• 2 tablespoons of brown sugar
• 1 tablespoon of apple cider vinegar
• 1 teaspoon of smoked paprika
• Salt and pepper to taste

Method of Preparation:

1. Start by setting your oven to 375°F.

2. In a skillet over medium heat, warm the olive oil. Around 5-7 minutes later, add the minced garlic and onion dice and continue to sauté until aromatic.

3. Add your can of rinsed and drained beans to the skillet along with the onions and garlic. To blend, stir.

4. Combine the tomato sauce, molasses, brown sugar, apple cider vinegar, smoked paprika, salt, and pepper in a different bowl.

5. After adding the sauce to the beans in the skillet, stir everything together thoroughly.

6. Put the bean mixture in a baking dish and heat the oven to 350 degrees for 30 to 35 minutes, or until the sauce is bubbly and thick.

7. Remove the baked beans from the oven and let them cool for a few minutes before serving.

By utilizing various types of beans or including extra ingredients like bacon or diced tomatoes, baked beans and other legumes can be tailored to your personal preferences in terms of flavor. By altering the amounts of molasses and smoked paprika, you may also change the dish's sweetness and smokiness.

A substantial and nutritious side dish that goes well with a variety of main meals is baked beans and lentils. They are a wonderful choice for weight gain diets since they are a great source of protein and fiber. Try this recipe for a satisfying and nourishing side dish that will leave you feeling energized.

Creamy Mashed Potatoes And Sweet Potatoes

Traditional side dishes like creamy mashed potatoes and sweet potatoes can be a terrific addition to a diet plan for weight gain. They are not only satisfying and delicious, but they are also a great source of vitamins and fiber. Here's a how-to for cooking sweet potatoes and creamy mashed potatoes:

Ingredients:

•4-6 potatoes (a mix of russet and sweet potatoes is ideal)
•1/4 cup of butter
•1/4 cup of heavy cream or milk
•Salt and pepper to taste

Method of Preparation:

1. Peel the potatoes, then slice them into big pieces. To get rid of extra starch, rinse them in cold water.

2. Fill a big pot with enough cold water to cover the potatoes. The potatoes should be cooked in boiling water for 20 to 25 minutes, or until they are fork-tender.

3. After the potatoes have been rinsed, add them back to the pot.

4. Add the potatoes to the pot along with the butter and heavy cream or milk. The potatoes should be smooth and creamy after being mashed using a potato masher or an electric mixer.

5. To taste, add salt and pepper to the mashed potatoes.

6. As a side dish, serve the hot mashed potatoes with your main course.

You can personalize creamy mashed potatoes and sweet potatoes to your preferences by including extras like cheese, chives, or garlic. Also, you can change the mashed potatoes' consistency by varying the amount of heavy cream or milk used.

Although they can contain a lot of carbohydrates, potatoes are also a fantastic source of fiber and vital nutrients like vitamin C and potassium. Your diet's calorie and nutritional requirements for weight gain can be met by including potatoes in moderation. So watch your portion sizes and combine your intake of potatoes with other nutrient-dense foods.

Mac And Cheese Variations

Many people enjoy mac and cheese, a traditional comfort food, and there are endless varieties of this recipe that you may try to change things up. Here are three different ways to prepare mac and cheese as a side dish:

Classic Mac and Cheese

Ingredients:

- 1 pound elbow macaroni
- 4 tablespoons butter
- 4 tablespoons flour
- 2 cups milk
- 1/2 teaspoon salt
- 1/4 teaspoon black pepper
- 2 cups shredded cheddar cheese

Method of Preparation:

1. Prepare the elbow macaroni as directed on the package.

2. Melt the butter in a different saucepan over medium heat. Blend in the flour after adding it.

3. Continue whisking as you gradually add the milk to the butter and flour mixture. Sauté for about 5 minutes, or until the mixture thickens.

4. Season the milk mixture with salt and black pepper.

5. Stir the milk mixture with the cheddar cheese until it has melted and the sauce is smooth.

6. Pour the cooked macaroni into the cheese sauce after draining. Mix the macaroni and cheese sauce together until well-coated.

Bacon and Jalapeño Mac and Cheese

Ingredients:

• 1 pound elbow macaroni
• 4 tablespoons butter
• 4 tablespoons flour
• 2 cups milk
• 1/2 teaspoon salt
• 1/4 teaspoon black pepper
• 2 cups shredded cheddar cheese
• 4 slices bacon, cooked and crumbled
• 2 jalapeños, seeded and diced

Method of Preparation:

1. Make the elbow macaroni according to the directions on the package.

2. Melt the butter over medium heat in a different saucepan. Whisk until smooth after adding the flour.

3. While continuously whisking the butter and flour mixture, gradually add the milk.

About 5 minutes of cooking should thicken the mixture.

4. Season the milk mixture with black pepper and salt.

5. Stir the cheddar cheese until it has melted and the sauce is smooth before adding it to the milk mixture.

6. Include the diced jalapenos and cooked, crumbled bacon in the cheese sauce.

7. Drain the macaroni that has been cooked, then stir it into the cheese sauce. The cheese sauce must be thoroughly mixed into the pasta.

Butternut Squash Mac and Cheese

Ingredients:

- 1 pound elbow macaroni
- 4 tablespoons butter
- 4 tablespoons flour

- 2 cups milk
- 1/2 teaspoon salt
- 1/4 teaspoon black pepper
- 2 cups shredded cheddar cheese
- 1 cup cooked and mashed butternut squash

Method of Preparation:

1. Make the elbow macaroni according to the directions on the package.

2. Melt the butter over medium heat in a different saucepan. Whisk until smooth after adding the flour.

3. While continuously whisking the butter and flour mixture, gradually add the milk. About 5 minutes of cooking should thicken the mixture.

4. Season the milk mixture with black pepper and salt.

5. Stir the milk mixture before adding the butternut squash and cheddar cheese.

Make sure the cheese is melted and the sauce is smooth.

6. After draining, add the cooked macaroni to the cheese sauce. The cheese sauce must be thoroughly mixed into the pasta.

These three variations of mac and cheese are just a few examples of the endless possibilities when it comes to this classic dish.

Garlic Bread And Rolls

Garlic bread and rolls are a simple and tasty side dish that can be served with a variety of main courses, from pasta dishes to soups and stews. Here's a recipe for homemade garlic bread and rolls that are sure to please your taste buds.

Ingredients:

•1 pound pizza dough (store-bought or homemade)

- 4 tablespoons unsalted butter, melted
- 4 cloves garlic, minced
- 1/4 teaspoon salt
- 1/4 teaspoon black pepper
- 1/4 teaspoon dried oregano
- 1/4 teaspoon dried parsley
- 1/4 teaspoon dried basil
- 1/2 cup grated Parmesan cheese

Method of preparation:

1. Set your oven to 400 degrees Fahrenheit.

2. Make 12 equal balls out of the pizza dough by dividing it into equal portions. They should be put on a parchment paper-lined baking sheet.

3. Combine the oregano, parsley, basil, oregano, salt, and black pepper in a small bowl with the melted butter.

4. Ensure that the dough balls are evenly covered with the garlic butter mixture by brushing it on top.

5. Cover the tops of the dough balls with grated Parmesan cheese.

6. Place the preheated oven on the lowest setting and bake the garlic rolls for 12 to 15 minutes, or until golden brown.

7. Prepare the garlic bread and bake the rolls simultaneously. A loaf of Italian bread should be split lengthwise.

8. Evenly cover the tops of the bread halves with the garlic butter mixture by brushing it on.

9. Top the bread halves with freshly grated Parmesan cheese.

10. Spread the garlic bread out on a baking sheet covered with parchment paper and bake it for 10 to 12 minutes, or until it turns golden brown, in the preheated oven.

11. Take the rolls and garlic bread out of the oven, and allow them to cool before serving.

Any dinner would be enhanced by these garlic rolls and toast. Garlic, herbs, and Parmesan cheese together will definitely make your taste buds happy.

Homemade Sauces And Dips

Your meals can be enhanced with flavor and nutrition by using homemade sauces and dips. They can be used as a sauce for meat, fish, or pasta dishes as well as a dip for vegetables, chips, or toast. The following recipe makes three different homemade sauces and dips that are great for weight gain and will definitely please your palate.

Avocado Dip

Ingredients:

- 2 ripe avocados
- 1/2 cup plain Greek yogurt
- 1 clove garlic, minced
- 1/4 teaspoon salt
- 1/4 teaspoon black pepper
- Juice of 1/2 lime

Method of Preparation:

1. Halve the avocados, scoop out the flesh into a bowl after removing the pit.

2. Fill the bowl with the Greek yogurt, lime juice, salt, black pepper, and minced garlic.

3. To make the dip smooth, mash the ingredients with a fork or potato masher.

4. Prior to serving, the dip should be chilled in the fridge for at least 30 minutes.

Tomato Sauce

Ingredients:

• 2 tablespoons olive oil
• 1 onion, diced
• 2 cloves garlic, minced
• 1 can (28 ounces) crushed tomatoes
• 1 teaspoon salt
• 1/2 teaspoon black pepper
• 1/4 teaspoon dried oregano

• 1/4 teaspoon dried basil
• 1/4 teaspoon dried thyme

Method of Preparation:

1. In a pan over medium heat, warm the olive oil.

2. Add the minced garlic and onion to the pan, and cook until the onion is translucent and soft.

3. Add salt, black pepper, oregano, basil, and thyme to the saucepan and stir to combine.

4. Lower the heat to low and simmer the sauce for 15 to 20 minutes, stirring now and then.

5. Before serving, let the sauce cool slightly.

Hummus

Ingredients:

- 1 can (15 ounces) chickpeas, drained and rinsed
- 1/4 cup tahini
- 1/4 cup olive oil
- Juice of 1 lemon
- 2 cloves garlic, minced
- 1/2 teaspoon salt
- 1/2 teaspoon ground cumin

Method of Preparation:

1. Place the chickpeas, tahini, olive oil, lemon juice, minced garlic, salt, and cumin in a food processor.

2. Pulse the ingredients until they are well combined and the hummus is smooth.

3. If the hummus is too thick, add a tablespoon of water at a time until it reaches the desired consistency.

4. Chill the hummus in the refrigerator for at least 30 minutes before serving.

These homemade sauces and dips are easy to make and are a great way to add flavor and nutrition to your meals. They are perfect for weight gain because they are made with healthy ingredients that are high in protein and healthy fats. So the next time you're looking for a delicious and healthy side dish, give one of these homemade sauces and dips a try!

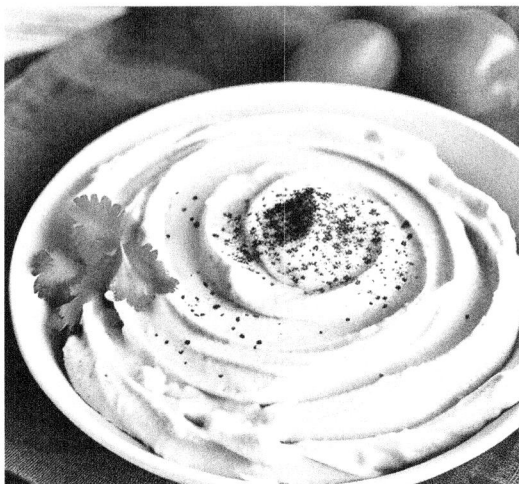

Hummus

CHAPTER SEVEN

Dessert

Protein-Packed Desserts For Weight Gain

Protein-packed desserts can be a great addition to your diet if you are looking to gain weight. These desserts are not only delicious but also packed with essential nutrients that can help you meet your daily protein needs. In this recipe, we will be making a protein-packed dessert that is easy to prepare and absolutely delicious.

Ingredients:

- 1 cup rolled oats
- 1 cup vanilla protein powder
- 1/2 cup almond butter
- 1/2 cup honey
- 1/2 cup dark chocolate chips
- 1/2 cup unsweetened coconut flakes

- 1/4 cup chopped almonds
- 1/4 cup dried cranberries
- 1/4 cup dried apricots
- 1/4 cup pumpkin seeds

Method of Preparation:

1. Preheat your oven to 350°F. Line an 8x8 inch baking dish with parchment paper.

2. In a large mixing bowl, combine the rolled oats and vanilla protein powder. Mix well.

3. In a small saucepan, heat the almond butter and honey over low heat until smooth and creamy. Stir constantly to prevent burning.

4. Pour the almond butter and honey mixture over the rolled oats and protein powder. Mix well until all the dry ingredients are coated.

5. Add the dark chocolate chips, unsweetened coconut flakes, chopped almonds, dried cranberries, dried apricots, and pumpkin seeds to the bowl. Mix well.

6. Pour the mixture into the prepared baking dish. Use a spatula to press down firmly and evenly.

7. Bake for 15-20 minutes, or until the edges are golden brown.

8. Remove from the oven and let it cool completely in the baking dish.

9. Once cooled, cut into squares and serve. Enjoy your delicious and protein-packed dessert.

This dessert is perfect for those who want to gain weight in a healthy and delicious way. It is also a great snack to have on hand when you need a quick energy boost. You can store these bars in an airtight container in the fridge for up to a week.

Cakes And Cupcakes

Cakes and cupcakes can be a delicious way to increase your calorie intake if you are looking to gain weight. However, most traditional cake and cupcake recipes are packed with sugar and unhealthy fats, making them a less than ideal option. In this recipe, we will be making a healthier version of cakes and cupcakes that are still tasty and indulgent, but also packed with nutritious ingredients.

For the Cakes

Ingredients

•2 cups almond flour
•1/2 cup coconut flour
•1/2 cup tapioca flour
•1/2 cup coconut sugar
•1 tsp baking powder
•1 tsp baking soda

- 1/2 tsp salt
- 1/2 cup coconut oil, melted
- 1 cup almond milk
- 3 eggs
- 1 tsp vanilla extract

For the frosting

- 1 cup raw cashews, soaked for at least 2 hours
- 1/4 cup coconut cream
- 2 tbsp maple syrup
- 1 tbsp coconut oil, melted
- 1 tsp vanilla extract

Method of Preparation:

1. Set your oven's temperature to 350°F. Make a parchment paper liner for a 9-inch cake pan.

2. Combine the almond flour, coconut flour, tapioca flour, coconut sugar, baking powder, baking soda, and salt in a sizable mixing bowl. Make a good mixture.

3. Combine the eggs, almond milk, melted coconut oil, and vanilla extract in a different bowl.

4. Add the wet ingredients to the dry ingredients and stir thoroughly to combine.

5. Transfer the batter to the ready cake pan, smoothing the top.

6. Bake for 25 to 30 minutes, or until a toothpick inserted in the center of the cake comes out clean.

7. Allow the cake to fully cool before frosting.

8. Drain the soaked cashews and combine them with the coconut cream, maple syrup, melted coconut oil, and vanilla extract in a high-speed blender to make the frosting. Mix until creamy and smooth.

9. After the cake has cooled, cover the top with the frosting.

10. To make cupcakes, use the same recipe, but instead of using a cake pan, pour the batter into lined cupcake molds. 18 to 20 minutes of baking.

For those who wish to indulge in a sweet treat while still eating healthily, this cake and cupcake recipe is a perfect choice. These treats are loaded with protein and good fats thanks to ingredients like almond flour and coconut sugar.

Pies And Tarts

Pies and tarts are traditional treats that go well with any meal. Traditional pie and tart recipes, however, may be laden with harmful fats and sugar. With this recipe, we'll create a healthier pie and tart that tastes just as good and is brimming with wholesome ingredients.

For the crust

Ingredients:

- 1 cup almond flour
- 1 cup oat flour
- 1/4 cup coconut oil, melted
- 2 tbsp maple syrup
- 1/2 tsp salt

For the filling

- 2 cups mixed berries (strawberries, blueberries, raspberries, etc.)
- 1/4 cup coconut sugar
- 1 tbsp cornstarch
- 1 tbsp lemon juice
- 1/2 tsp vanilla extract

For the topping

- 1/2 cup rolled oats

•1/2 cup chopped nuts (walnuts, pecans, almonds, etc.)
•1/4 cup coconut sugar
•1/4 cup coconut oil, melted
•1/2 tsp cinnamon

Method of Preparation:

1. Set the oven to 350°F.

2. Combine the melted coconut oil, oat flour, salt, maple syrup, and almond flour in a mixing bowl to make the crust. Everything should be thoroughly blended after mixing.

3. Using either a 9-inch pie plate or several smaller tart pans, press the mixture into the pans, making sure the crust is distributed evenly.

4. Combine the mixed berries, cornstarch, lemon juice, vanilla extract, coconut sugar, and corn syrup in a bowl to make the filling.

5. Spoon the mixture into the crust.

6. In a mixing bowl, combine the cinnamon, coconut sugar, melted coconut oil, chopped nuts, and rolled oats to make the topping. Blend thoroughly.

7. Drizzle the berry filling with the topping.

8. Bake the pie for 30-35 minutes, or until the crust is golden brown and the filling is bubbling.

9. Before cutting and serving the pie or tart, allow it to cool completely.

For those who wish to indulge in dessert while still eating well, this recipe for pie and tart is a terrific choice. These treats are loaded with fiber and good fats thanks to ingredients like coconut sugar and almond flour. The mixed fruit filling is also chock-full of vitamins and antioxidants.

Cheesecake And Pudding Variations

Cheesecake and pudding are two classic dessert options that are both creamy and decadent. However, they can be high in calories and sugar, making them a less than ideal option for those looking to gain weight in a healthy way. In this recipe, we will be making a healthier version of cheesecake and pudding that are high in protein and packed with nutritious ingredients.

For the cheesecake

Ingredients:

- 2 cups Greek yogurt
- 2 cups cream cheese, softened
- 1/2 cup honey
- 1 tsp vanilla extract
- 4 large eggs

For the pudding:

- 2 cups almond milk
- 1/2 cup chia seeds

•1/4 cup honey
•1 tsp vanilla extract
•1/4 tsp salt

Method of Preparation:

1. Preheat your oven to 325°F.

2. To make the cheesecake, beat the Greek yogurt, cream cheese, honey, and vanilla extract together in a large mixing bowl until smooth.

3. Beat in the eggs, one at a time, making sure each egg is fully incorporated before adding the next one.

4. Pour the mixture into a greased 9-inch springform pan.

5. Bake for 45-50 minutes or until the cheesecake is set.

6. Let the cheesecake cool to room temperature before refrigerating for at least 2 hours.

7. To make the pudding, combine the almond milk, chia seeds, honey, vanilla extract, and salt in a mixing bowl.

8. Whisk everything together until well combined.

9. Let the mixture sit for at least 10 minutes, whisking occasionally until it has thickened to a pudding-like consistency.

10. Once the pudding has set, serve it topped with fresh berries, chopped nuts, or your favorite toppings.

This cheesecake and pudding recipe is a great way to indulge in a sweet treat while still maintaining a healthy diet. Greek yogurt and cream cheese are both high in protein, making this cheesecake a great option for those looking to build muscle. Chia seeds in the pudding add an extra boost of protein and fiber, helping to keep you full and satisfied. Plus, with natural sweeteners like honey and vanilla extract, these desserts are much healthier than traditional options.

Ice Cream And Frozen Yogurt Variations

Ice cream and frozen yogurt are two classic dessert options that are perfect for any occasion. However, traditional ice cream and frozen yogurt recipes can be high in sugar and unhealthy fats. In this recipe, we will be making a healthier version of ice cream and frozen yogurt that are just as delicious but also packed with nutritious ingredients.

For the ice cream:

Ingredients:

•2 cups coconut cream
•1/4 cup honey

- 1 tsp vanilla extract
- 1/4 tsp salt
- 1/2 cup mix-ins (chopped nuts, chocolate chips, fruit, etc.)

For the frozen yogurt:

- 2 cups Greek yogurt
- 1/4 cup honey
- 1 tsp vanilla extract
- 1/2 cup mix-ins (chopped nuts, fruit, etc.)

Method of Preparation:

1. To make the ice cream, combine the coconut cream, honey, vanilla extract, and salt in a mixing bowl. Mix everything thoroughly until it is all combined.

2. Put the mixture in an ice cream maker and churn it as directed by the manufacturer.

3. Add your preferred mix-ins to the ice cream after it has thickened and churn for a few more minutes to fully incorporate them.

4. Before serving, place the ice cream in a freezer-safe container and freeze for at least two hours.

5. In a mixing bowl, combine the Greek yogurt, honey, and vanilla extract to make the frozen yogurt. Stir everything thoroughly until it is all mixed.

6. Add in your choice of mix-ins and mix until they are well incorporated.

7. Transfer the mixture to an ice cream maker and churn according to the manufacturer's instructions.

8. Once the frozen yogurt has thickened, transfer it to a freezer-safe container and freeze for at least 2 hours before serving.

These ice cream and frozen yogurt recipes are a great option for those who want to indulge in a sweet treat while still maintaining a healthy diet. Coconut cream in the ice cream recipe is a great source of healthy fats, while Greek yogurt in the frozen yogurt recipe is high in protein.

Fruit Crumbles And Cobblers

Fruit crumbles and cobblers are classic desserts that are easy to make and perfect for any occasion. However, traditional recipes can be high in sugar and lacking in nutritional value. In this recipe, we will be making a healthier version of fruit crumbles and cobblers that are packed with nutritious ingredients and perfect for those looking to gain weight in a healthy way.

For the filling

Ingredients:

•4 cups of fresh or frozen fruit (peaches, berries, apples, etc.)
•1/4 cup honey
•1 tbsp cornstarch

•1 tsp vanilla extract
•1/4 tsp salt

For the topping:
•1 cup oats
•1/2 cup almond flour
•1/4 cup chopped nuts (pecans, almonds, etc.)
•1/4 cup honey
•1/4 cup melted coconut oil
•1 tsp vanilla extract
•1/4 tsp salt

Method of Preparation:

1. Preheat your oven to 375°F.

2. To make the filling, combine the fruit, honey, cornstarch, vanilla extract, and salt in a mixing bowl.

3. Transfer the fruit mixture to a 9-inch baking dish.

4. To make the topping, combine the oats, almond flour, chopped nuts, honey, coconut oil, vanilla extract, and salt in a mixing bowl. Stir everything up thoroughly after mixing.

5. Sprinkle the topping evenly over the fruit mixture.

6. Bake for 35-40 minutes or until the topping is golden brown and the fruit is bubbling.

7. Let the crumble or cobbler cool for a few minutes before serving.

This fruit crumble or cobbler recipe is a great way to indulge in a sweet treat while still maintaining a healthy diet. Fruit is packed with vitamins, minerals, and fiber, making this dessert a nutritious option. Plus, with natural sweeteners like honey and vanilla extract, this recipe is much healthier than traditional options. The use of almond flour and coconut oil in the topping provides healthy fats, while the use of nuts adds an extra boost of protein.

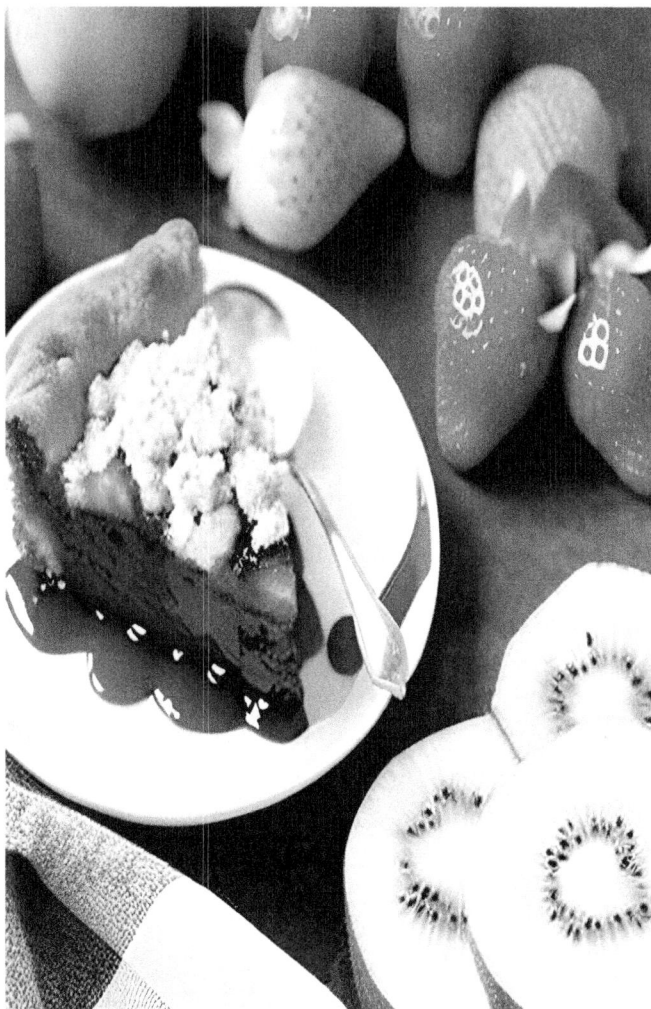

Fruit Crumbles And Cobblers

CHAPTER EIGHT

Meal Planning and Preparation Tips

Tips For Efficient Meal Planning

Meal planning is a crucial part of gaining weight, as it allows you to stay on track with your nutritional goals and ensure that you are consuming enough calories and nutrients to support muscle growth. However, for beginners, meal planning can be overwhelming and challenging. In this writing, we will provide some tips for efficient meal planning to help beginners achieve their weight gain goals.

Set Realistic Goals:
The first step in efficient meal planning is to set realistic goals. You should have a clear understanding of your weight gain goals, whether it's to gain a certain amount of weight, build muscle mass, or improve your

overall health. Once you have established your goals, you can work on creating a meal plan that aligns with your needs.

Calculate Your Caloric Needs:
To gain weight, you need to consume more calories than you burn. Therefore, it is essential to calculate your daily caloric needs. You can use online calculators or consult a dietitian to determine your daily caloric intake. Once you have this number, you can start planning your meals accordingly.

Focus on Nutrient-Dense Foods:
When planning your meals, focus on nutrient-dense foods such as lean proteins, complex carbohydrates, healthy fats, and fruits and vegetables. These foods provide your body with the essential nutrients it needs to build muscle mass and support overall health.

Plan Your Meals in Advance:
Planning your meals in advance is key to efficient meal planning. Take the time to plan your meals for the week ahead, including breakfast, lunch, dinner, and snacks. This will help you stay on track with your nutritional goals and ensure that you have the necessary ingredients on hand.

Keep it Simple:
When starting out with meal planning, it is best to keep it simple. Start with basic meals that you enjoy and gradually add more variety as you become more comfortable with meal planning. You do not need to create elaborate meals to achieve your weight gain goals.

Prep Your Meals in Advance:
Prepping your meals in advance can save you time and ensure that you always have healthy meals on hand. Set aside a few hours each week to prepare your meals for the week ahead. This can include cooking your proteins, chopping your vegetables, and

portioning out your snacks.

Be Flexible:
Finally, it is essential to be flexible with your meal planning. Life can be unpredictable, and there may be times when you are unable to stick to your meal plan. It is okay to deviate from your plan occasionally. The key is to get back on track as soon as possible and continue working towards your goals.

In conclusion, efficient meal planning is essential for weight gain beginners. By setting realistic goals, calculating your caloric needs, focusing on nutrient-dense foods, planning your meals in advance, keeping it simple, prepping your meals in advance, and being flexible, you can create a meal plan that aligns with your needs and helps you achieve your weight gain goals.

How To Prep Meals In Advance

Meal prepping is a key component of any successful weight gain journey. By prepping your meals in advance, you can ensure that you have healthy, nutrient-dense meals on hand at all times, which can help you stay on track with your weight gain goals. In this writing, we will discuss some tips on how to prep meals in advance for weight gain beginners.

Plan Your Meals:
The first step in meal prepping is to plan your meals. Take some time to sit down and decide what meals you will be eating for the week. This will help you determine what ingredients you will need and how much of each.

Shop for Ingredients:
Once you have your meal plan, it's time to go grocery shopping. Make a list of all the ingredients you need, and make sure to include plenty of nutrient-dense foods such

as lean proteins, complex carbohydrates, healthy fats, and fruits and vegetables.

Cook in Batches:
When prepping your meals, it's best to cook in batches. This means cooking multiple servings of each meal at once. Not only will this save you time, but it will also ensure that you have enough food to last throughout the week.

Invest in Storage Containers:
Investing in storage containers is essential for meal prepping. Choose containers that are microwave and dishwasher safe, and make sure they are the right size for your portions. This will help keep your meals fresh and organized.

Portion Out Your Meals:
When prepping your meals, it's important to portion them out properly. Use a food scale or measuring cups to ensure that you are getting the right amount of each ingredient.

This will help you stay on track with your caloric goals.

Label Your Containers:
A great approach to maintain organization is to label your containers. On the label, provide the meal's name, the date it was prepared, and any applicable cooking instructions. This will make it simple to grab and go in a hurry.

Store your meals properly:
Maintaining proper storage is essential for keeping your food fresh. Depending on how soon you intend to eat them, store your meals in the refrigerator or freezer. To avoid deterioration, be sure to store them in airtight containers.

Mix it Up:
Finally, it's important to mix up your meals. Eating the same thing every day can get boring, so try to incorporate different flavors and textures into your meals. This will help keep you motivated and excited about your

weight gain journey.

Time-Saving Cooking Techniques For Weight Gain

When it comes to gaining weight, one of the biggest challenges is finding the time to cook and prepare healthy meals. However, there are several time-saving cooking techniques that can help you stay on track with your weight gain goals, even when you're short on time.

Batch Cooking:
Batch cooking is one of the most effective time-saving techniques for weight gain. This involves cooking large batches of food in advance, and then storing them in the fridge or freezer for later use. By cooking in bulk, you can save time on meal prep throughout the week, while still ensuring that you have healthy, nutrient-dense meals on hand at all times.

Slow Cooking:
Another great time-saving cooking technique for weight gain is slow cooking. This involves using a slow cooker or crockpot to cook your meals over several hours. Slow cooking allows you to prepare large batches of food with minimal effort, while still ensuring that the flavors are rich and complex. Plus, slow cooking can be a great way to tenderize tougher cuts of meat, making them easier to digest and more nutrient-dense.

One-Pot Meals:
One-pot meals are another great time-saving cooking technique for weight gain. These meals involve cooking all of your ingredients in a single pot or pan, which means less time spent washing dishes and more time spent enjoying your meal. One-pot meals can be made with a variety of ingredients, from pasta and rice to beans and vegetables, making them a versatile and nutritious option for weight gain.

Meal Prep Kits:
Meal prep kits are a convenient and time-saving option for weight gain. These kits typically include pre-portioned ingredients and recipes, which means all you have to do is follow the instructions and cook the meal. Meal prep kits can be a great option for busy individuals who don't have time to plan and shop for ingredients, while still ensuring that you have healthy, nutrient-dense meals on hand.

Multi-Tasking:
Finally, one of the best ways to save time in the kitchen is by multi-tasking. For example, while you're waiting for your water to boil for pasta, you can chop up vegetables or marinate meat for later use. By multi-tasking and planning your cooking process in advance, you can save time and ensure that your meals are ready when you need them.

In conclusion, time-saving cooking techniques can be incredibly helpful for individuals looking to gain weight. By using techniques such as batch cooking, slow cooking, one-pot meals, meal prep kits, and multi-tasking, you can save time in the kitchen while still ensuring that you have healthy, nutrient-dense meals on hand at all times. With a little planning and preparation, you can achieve your weight gain goals while still maintaining a busy lifestyle.

Creative Ways To Add Healthy Carbs and Fats To Your Meals

When it comes to gaining weight, it's important to focus on consuming nutrient-dense foods that are high in healthy carbohydrates and fats. However, it can be challenging to come up with creative ways to incorporate these foods into your meals. Here are some ideas for adding healthy carbs and fats to your meals in delicious and creative ways.

Add Avocado:
Avocado is a fantastic source of healthy fats and can be easily incorporated into a variety

of meals. Try adding sliced avocado to your morning toast, or use it as a topping for salads, tacos, or sandwiches. You can also blend avocado into smoothies or use it as a base for homemade salad dressings.

Incorporate Nut Butters:
Nut butters, such as peanut butter or almond butter, are a great source of healthy fats and can be added to a variety of meals. Spread nut butter on toast or use it as a dip for fruit. You can also mix nut butter into oatmeal or yogurt for a delicious and filling breakfast.

Use Healthy Oils:
Healthy oils, such as olive oil, coconut oil, or avocado oil, are a great source of healthy fats and can be used in cooking or as a dressing for salads. Try roasting vegetables in olive oil or using coconut oil to fry up some sweet potato fries.

Incorporate Grains:
Whole grains, such as brown rice, quinoa, or barley, are an excellent source of healthy

carbohydrates and can be used in a variety of meals. Try adding cooked grains to salads or stir-fry dishes. You can also use grains as a base for a hearty grain bowl or as a side dish to accompany a protein source.

Use Sweet Potatoes:
Sweet potatoes are an excellent source of healthy carbs and can be incorporated into a variety of meals. Try roasting sweet potatoes and adding them to salads or use them as a base for a breakfast bowl. You can also mash sweet potatoes and use them as a healthy alternative to traditional mashed potatoes.

Incorporate Legumes:
Legumes, such as beans or lentils, are an excellent source of healthy carbohydrates and can be used in a variety of meals. Try adding beans or lentils to soups, stews, or chili for a filling and nutritious meal. You can also use legumes as a base for a vegetarian burger or add them to a salad for extra protein and fiber.

With a little experimentation, you can find the perfect balance of healthy carbs and fats to keep you feeling full and energized throughout the day.

Creative Ways To Incorporate Healthy Fats Into Your Sweets

It may seem counterintuitive to include healthy fats in your sweets, but doing so can be a terrific way to give your favorite treats more flavor, texture, and nutrition. Here are some inventive methods for including healthy fats in desserts:

Utilize Nut Butters: Nut butters, such almond or peanut butter, are an excellent source of good fats and may be included into a number of treats. For more flavor and richness, try incorporating nut butter into your favorite brownie or cookie dough. Moreover, nut butter can be used as an ice cream topping or a filling for homemade chocolates.

Avocado should be added because it is a fruit that works well in both savory and sweet meals. Avocado can be used in baking delicacies like cakes and cupcakes in place of butter or oil. A tasty and healthy chocolate mousse may be made by combining avocado with cocoa powder, honey, and almond milk.

Usage Coconut Oil: Coconut oil is a fantastic source of healthy fats and may be used in baking recipes in place of butter or oil. To add flavor and richness to your favorite cookie or brownie recipe, try incorporating coconut oil. Also, you can use coconut oil to create your own granola bars or energy bites.

Including Nuts and Seeds: A variety of desserts can benefit from the addition of nuts and seeds, which are a fantastic source of healthy fats.To give your favorite cake or muffin recipe more texture and crunch, try adding chopped nuts or seeds. Also, you can prepare your own nut or seed butter to put on toast or as a filling for baked items.

Employ Dark Chocolate: A variety of desserts can benefit from the addition of dark chocolate, which is a fantastic source of antioxidants and healthy fats. For a treat that is both healthful and decadent, try melting dark chocolate and dipping almonds or fresh fruit in it. Also, you can use dark chocolate to garnish yogurt or oatmeal or to make your own truffles.

Greek yogurt can be used in place of butter or oil in baking recipes and is a fantastic source of protein.To add moisture and nutrition to your favorite cake or muffin recipe, try incorporating Greek yogurt. Greek yogurt can also be used to create a delicious and healthy icing for cakes or cupcakes.

In order to gain weight, there are a variety of inventive ways to add healthy fats to your sweets. You may enjoy decadent desserts and yet obtain the nutrients your body requires by combining foods like nut butters, avocado, coconut oil, nuts and seeds, dark chocolate, and Greek yogurt into your baked goods. You may find the ideal ratio of healthy fats to keep you full and energized with a little testing.

Common Concerns And Questions About Weight Gain

Whether it's for health reasons, to enhance sports performance, or just to feel more confident in one's looks, weight gain is a prevalent worry for many people. The following are some typical worries and queries regarding weight gain:

How much should I eat to gain weight?

Your height, weight, age, and degree of activity, among other things, all affect how much weight you should gain. A healthy pace of weight increase is typically between 0.5 and 1 pound each week. But, it's crucial to speak with a medical expert to establish a healthy weight gain target that is appropriate for your particular circumstances.

What are some wholesome ways to put on weight?

Eating a balanced diet with an emphasis on nutrient-dense foods, such as fruits, vegetables, whole grains, lean meats, and healthy fats, is one good method to gain weight. To increase muscle mass, it's also crucial to engage in regular physical exercise like weightlifting or resistance training.

Is it possible to gain weight without consuming junk food?

Absolutely, you can gain weight without consuming junk food. A diet high in whole, nutrient-dense foods is actually more likely to encourage healthy weight gain and enhance overall health. Whole grains and fruits are healthy sources of carbs that can provide your body the energy it needs to grow muscle.while the building blocks for muscular growth can be found in lean proteins and healthy fats.

How can I tell if I'm growing fat or muscle?

Monitor your body composition over time to discover whether you're growing muscle or fat. There are several ways to do this, including documenting body measurements, taking progress photos, and calculating body fat percentage. It's also crucial to remember that weight increase can consist of both muscle and fat, proving that it's not always an either/or choice.

What if I don't get any outcomes?

If your weight gain attempts aren't producing the desired results, it could be time to reconsider your strategy.To make sure you're ingesting enough calories and exercising enough to promote weight gain, think about tracking your eating and exercise routines. A licensed dietician or healthcare expert can help you create a customized plan that takes into consideration your particular needs and objectives.

There are many different aspects to take into account while discussing the topic of weight increase. You may encourage healthy weight gain and enhance overall health by putting a focus on nutrient-dense diets and regular physical activity. It is always best to speak with a healthcare expert or registered dietitian if you are worried about or have questions regarding weight gain so that you can create a custom strategy that is effective for you.

Tips For Overcoming Weight Gain Plateaus

Though they can be upsetting and demoralizing, weight gain plateaus are a common aspect of the process of gaining weight. The following advice can assist you in overcoming weight gain plateaus and advancing toward your objectives:

Increased Calorie Intake: You may need to up your calorie intake if you've reached a weight growth plateau. Your body may have adjusted to the calories you consume now, so boosting them may help rev up your metabolism and promote muscle growth. To avoid accumulating too much fat, it's crucial to do this gradually and track your development.

Monitor Your Macros: One way to break through weight gain plateaus is by keeping track of your macronutrient consumption. Make sure you're consuming enough protein to aid in the growth of your muscles, and modify your carbohydrate and fat intake as necessary. To maximize your nutrient intake, you might also want to think about adjusting the frequency or time of your meals.

Change Your Workouts: Changing up your exercise regimen can aid in breaking through weight-gain plateaus. To push your muscles in different ways, try introducing new exercises or altering the intensity or length of your workouts. By doing so, you can promote muscle growth and stop your body from adjusting to your regimen.

Increase Your Protein Intake: As protein is necessary for muscle building, boosting your protein consumption can assist you in breaking through weight-gain plateaus. Increase your consumption of lean meats, fish, eggs, dairy products, and plant-based sources of protein like beans and nuts. You might also think about using protein supplements in your diet, like whey protein powder.

Get Enough Sleep: Sleeping sufficiently is important to break through weight gain plateaus since it promotes muscular regeneration and growth. Make sure you get adequate sleep, and give your muscles time to recuperate by taking rest days in between workouts. Your success may be hampered by weariness and injuries brought on by overtraining.

Contact a Professional: If you're having trouble breaking through a weight gain plateau, think about seeking expert advice. A nutritionist or personal trainer can assist you in developing a tailored strategy that takes into consideration your particular objectives, way of life, and preferences. Also, they can offer encouragement and support to keep you on track.

In conclusion, weight gain plateaus might be discouraging, but they are a common occurrence during the process of gaining weight. You can get beyond weight gain plateaus and keep moving forward toward your objectives by increasing your calorie intake, monitoring your macronutrients, mixing up your workouts, consuming more protein, getting enough rest, and talking to a specialist. You'll eventually get through your plateau and reach your ideal weight if you're persistent and patient.

Strategies For Maintaining A Healthy Weight

For general health and well-being, it's crucial to maintain a healthy weight. But, in a world where we are continuously exposed to poor food alternatives and a sedentary lifestyle, it can be difficult to maintain a healthy weight. The following are some tips for keeping a healthy weight:

Make healthy eating a habit

One of the most effective ways to maintain a healthy weight is to make healthy eating a habit. This means choosing whole, nutrient-dense foods over processed and junk foods. Aim to consume a variety of fruits, vegetables, whole grains, lean proteins, and healthy fats in your diet. It's also important to be mindful of portion sizes, as overeating can contribute to weight gain.

Stay active
To keep your weight within a healthy range, you must engage in regular physical activity. Try to work out for at least 30 minutes, most days of the week, at a moderate level. These can involve exercises like cycling, strength training, walking, and jogging. Discover activities you like to do and incorporate them into your routine on a regular basis.

Remain hydrated.
Keeping a healthy weight requires drinking adequate water. Dehydration not only makes it easier to overeat, but water also aids in toxin removal and supports a healthy digestive system. Try to consume eight glasses of water a day or more if you exercise frequently or live in a warm region.

Reduce stress
Stress can increase body cortisol levels, which can lead to weight gain. Overeating and the development of belly fat may result from this. Use relaxation methods like yoga, meditation, or deep breathing to control your

tension. Take part in enjoyable stress-relieving activities, such as spending time in nature or listening to music.

Get enough rest.

A healthy weight can only be sustained with adequate sleep. Hormones that control metabolism and hunger can be disturbed by a lack of sleep, which can cause overeating and weight gain. To encourage sound sleeping habits, aim for 7-8 hours of sleep per night and create a consistent bedtime routine.

Keep your word.

A strong tool for maintaining a healthy weight is accountability. This can involve keeping a journal of your dietary intake and exercise routines, participating in support groups, or consulting a doctor or trained dietitian. Having a regular check-in partner can assist you in staying on track and making good decisions.

7-Days Weight Gain Meal Plan

Here is a 7-day meal plan for weight gain that includes breakfast, snack, lunch, dinner, side, and dessert recipes:

Day 1

Breakfast: High-calorie smoothie made with banana, peanut butter, chocolate protein powder, and almond milk.

Snack: Homemade protein bars with chocolate chips and almonds.

Lunch: Grilled chicken salad with mixed greens, avocado, cherry tomatoes, and balsamic vinaigrette.

Dinner: Beef stir-fry with broccoli, carrots, and brown rice.

Side: Roasted sweet potatoes with garlic and rosemary.

Dessert: Chocolate protein pudding with sliced strawberries.

Day 2

Breakfast: Pancakes topped with sliced banana, walnuts, and maple syrup.

Snack: Trail mix with mixed nuts, dried fruit, and dark chocolate.

Lunch: Turkey and avocado sandwich with whole-grain bread, lettuce, and tomato.

Dinner: Baked salmon with lemon and herbs, served with quinoa and steamed asparagus.

Side: Garlic bread made with whole-grain bread.

Dessert: Blueberry crumble with oatmeal topping and vanilla ice cream.

Day 3

Breakfast: Oatmeal with peanut butter, honey, and sliced bananas.

Snack: Smoothie bowl made with Greek yogurt, mixed berries, and granola.

Lunch: Spaghetti carbonara with bacon, eggs, and Parmesan cheese.

Dinner: Beef chili with kidney beans, corn, and diced tomatoes.

Side: Baked beans with molasses and bacon.

Dessert: Apple pie with a whole-grain crust.

Day 4

Breakfast: Breakfast wrap with scrambled eggs, cheese, and spinach.

Snack: Homemade hummus with pita chips and sliced vegetables.

Lunch: Grilled chicken Caesar salad with whole-grain croutons and shaved Parmesan cheese.

Dinner: Grilled steak with roasted vegetables and baked potatoes.

Side: Creamy mashed potatoes with butter and sour cream.

Dessert: Chocolate cupcakes with vanilla frosting.

Day 5

Breakfast: Banana bread with almond butter.

Snack: Cheese and fruit plate with whole-grain crackers.

Lunch: Lentil soup with carrots, celery, and diced tomatoes.

Dinner: Chicken and vegetable stir-fry with brown rice.

Side: Grilled vegetables with balsamic glaze.

Dessert: Strawberry cheesecake with graham cracker crust.

Day 6

Breakfast: Waffles with mixed berries and whipped cream.

Snack: Popcorn with melted butter and grated Parmesan cheese.

Lunch: Tuna salad sandwich with whole-grain bread, lettuce, and tomato.

Dinner: Baked chicken parmesan with whole-grain pasta and marinara sauce.

Side: Grilled corn on the cob with garlic butter.

Dessert: Vanilla ice cream with caramel sauce.

Day 7

Breakfast: Breakfast casserole with eggs, sausage, and vegetables.

Snack: Yogurt bowl with granola and mixed berries.

Lunch: Vegetable and bean burrito with whole-grain tortilla.

Dinner: Grilled shrimp skewers with mixed vegetables and quinoa.

Side: Macaroni and cheese with breadcrumbs.

Dessert: Mixed berry tart with a whole-grain crust.

CONCLUSION

In conclusion, a beginner's weight gain cookbook can be a very helpful tool for people who want to eat more calories and acquire muscle mass. A weight gain cookbook can assist people in achieving their fitness and health objectives while fostering general health and wellbeing by offering recipes and meal plans that are full of nutrient-dense components.

A weight gain cookbook's recipes and advice can assist people in overcoming typical weight gain obstacles like meal planning and food preparation. A weight gain cookbook can assist people in achieving their macronutrient targets while advancing general health and wellness by providing innovative methods to combine nutritious carbs, fats, and proteins into meals.

A cookbook for weight gain can also provide people a sense of community and support as they start their weight-growth journey. A weight gain cookbook can help people take control of their health and fitness and reach their goals by providing advice on how to break through plateaus and keep a healthy weight.

Ultimately, anyone trying to up their caloric intake and add muscle mass will benefit from using a beginner's weight gain recipe. A weight gain cookbook can assist people in achieving their fitness and health objectives while enhancing general health and well-being by offering recipes, meal planning, and advice for overcoming typical obstacles connected to weight gain.

14-DAYS WEIGHT GAIN PLANNER

Days	Recipes	Remarks
1		
2		
3		

4		
5		
6		
7		

8		
9		
10		
11		

12		
13		
14		

Printed in Great Britain
by Amazon

26110927R00126